What are you full of? The answer to th......... life squeezes you. When something or so............. .... your control seeks to rob you of your hope or your joy. When Mary Naegeli was squeezed by cancer, what she's full of became evident. Grace and truth and honest pleading are what you will find in the raw and radically faithful writing of this gracious saint. If you've ever wondered how a person of faith can experience pain and find purpose, or give glory to God at the cellular and granular level, or if you just need to know the anchor really holds, these reflections are for you.

—Carmen LaBerge, radio host and author of *Speak the Truth:
How to Bring God Back into Every Conversation*

This highly personal and radically transparent memoir of Rev. Mary's physical and spiritual journey through "the valley of the shadow of death" with advanced lung cancer is informative, moving, and ultimately a call to discipleship through intimacy with Christ. Her honest realism and insightful biblical reflections provide encouragement and hope both for those suffering threatening illness and for those who walk alongside them as companions on the Way. I highly recommend this, both for its insight and for the gems of wisdom to help us on our own daily pilgrimage of life in the love of Christ. I was blessed and challenged in reading it.

—The Rev. Dr. Roberta Hestenes, pastor, former professor at
Fuller Seminary, and president of Eastern University

Breath is our life and our moment-by-moment hope: the breath of our lungs, the breath of others whom we love and who love us, the breath of living creatures. All this breath is derived from the ultimate source of all breath, the very *ruach*, or breath of God. Mary Naegeli's story of lung cancer draws us into the particularities of this especially insidious cancer and its physical, emotional, and spiritual taunts and tyrannies. It is a tale of the very stuff of life. Read it. Breathe deeply. You will be glad you did.

—Mark Labberton, president, Fuller Theological Seminary

How does one write a book that is both very personal and very helpful for others? With great care, the Rev. Dr. Mary Holder Naegeli has done just that. Mary's writing is clear, compelling, insightful, personal, faithful.

Deep Breathing journeys deeply through her lung cancer diagnosis and treatment, her feelings and insights, some fundamentals of Christian faith, and even the seasons of the church calendar. She manages capably to weave these strands together into a delightful and hopeful whole.

Whether one is staring down personal cancer, supporting a loved one in the journey, wondering what God is up to, or supplying spiritual care, this is an insightful resource.

—The Rev. James D. Berkley, pastor, writer, editor

One day you may receive unexpected news that turns your world upside down. How do you begin to navigate your new life—one now filled with loss, suffering, and pain? When pastor, musician, and creative thinker Mary Holder Naegeli was diagnosed with cancer, she merely veered down a new path on her life journey, which was already one of holding tight to the hand of Jesus. *Deep Breathing* is a brilliant and beautiful manifestation of how God's people can use a lifetime of spiritual deposits to guide the inevitable hard days. *What I need to know, I have in my possession already: a vision of life that is infused with joy, filled with the Spirit, empowered by God's grace, baited by good life-questions, and met with insatiable curiosity. I am going to keep living this life until God says, "Stop."* Follow Mary's journal, which so cleverly interweaves classic spiritual resources with everyday life experiences. And then please buy another copy for a gift—there are so many who need to learn to breathe in deeply the grace and mercy of our loving God.

—Lucinda Secrest McDowell,
author of *Soul Strong* and *Life-Giving Choices*

DEEP BREATHING

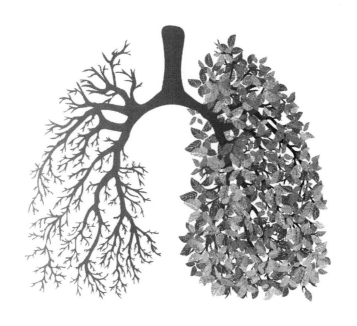

DEEP BREATHING

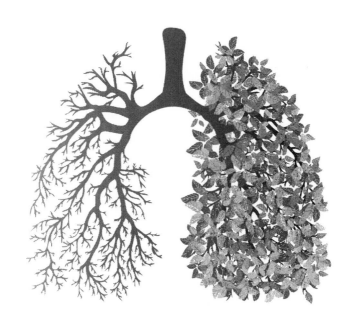

Finding Calm
amid Cancer Anxiety

REDEMPTION
PRESS

MARY HOLDER NAEGELI

Cover image / Igor Zubkov

Published by Redemption Press, PO Box 427, Enumclaw, WA 98022.

Toll-Free (844) 2REDEEM (273-3336)

Redemption Press is honored to present this title in partnership with the author. The views expressed or implied in this work are those of the author. Redemption Press provides our imprint seal representing design excellence, creative content, and high-quality production.

ISBN: 978-1-64645-119-7 (Paperback)
978-1-64645-120-3 (ePub)
978-1-64645-121-0 (Mobi)

Library of Congress Catalog Card Number: 2020909321

CONTENTS

EPIPHANY

LENT

EASTERTIDE

FOREWORD

M UCH LIKE BOTH MY PARENTS, I do not cry easily or often. I save my
tears for a quiet moment alone or perhaps a dark movie theater,
where no one can see me.

But on Monday, November 4, at 5:37 p.m., I opened an email from
my mother with the subject line "The biopsy report is in" and read: "No
good way to put this. The mass in my left lung is a cancerous tumor . . ."
And the tears began immediately, uncontrolled.

I was in the graduate reading room in the library of Seattle Pacific
University, where I attended seminary. Several other students were in the
room, completely oblivious to the news I had just received. *My mother has lung cancer.* Though the tears practically blinded me, I read on,
absorbing only a few words at a time: "stage III," "MRI," "oncologist,"
"radiation," "surgery." And that was when a sob escaped me. Mercifully,
everyone in the room was wearing headphones, and no one looked up.
I quickly packed my stuff and headed back to my house in Seattle (*two
states away from my parents!*). Unstoppable tears sprang out of me like a
sprinkler system. So when I opened the front door of my house and saw
my roommate working at the desk, I blurted, "It's stage three cancer!"
and nearly collapsed on the floor. Instinctively, my roommate jumped up
and enveloped me in a bear hug. I don't think she had ever seen me cry,
especially such an ugly cry as that.

Mom and Dad wanted to conference call with my sister and me that
evening, so when I felt like I had a little control of myself, I went to my

room to wait for the call. While waiting, I read the email again more carefully. "The surgeon said much better results are achieved by doing chemo and radiation first, and then whatever is left of the tumor is removed surgically . . ." Panic consumed me again. I paced around my room, breaking out into sobs periodically. *How could she possibly have lung cancer? She's never smoked a day in her life! What if she loses her hair? How will Dad be able to take care of her? Should I quit school? Will she . . . die?*

I read the email yet again, and this time landed on her last paragraph: "Your prayers and concern have already laid out a foundation of comfort and peace for me. I have every confidence that God will keep me calm, curious, and courageous for what lies ahead."

Calm, curious, and courageous? I asked myself. *Is that really an option?*

Clearly, my reaction to my mother's cancer could not be characterized by calmness, curiosity, or courage. But somehow, when I stopped to think about it for a moment, it made perfect sense that that was my mother's reaction. I grew up watching her pastor two congregations, teach classes, manage her household, and help me through my childhood struggles. She came to conflict calmly, even when I yelled at her as a teenager. She was curious about people and issues, delighting in everyday lessons and insights. And in situations when others might falter or cower, she stood her ground. She always came at things systematically, logically, and with integrity. Of course she would respond to cancer the same way!

As her child, it's easy for me to believe that she was always like that. Maybe some of these characteristics came from a God-given inborn nature, but she will tell you that she *learned* how to be calm, curious, and courageous with God's help. She will also tell you that you can too.

Dealing with cancer—whether as a patient, a caregiver, or a faraway family member—is not for the faint of heart. It can feel at times like the world is ending. When I found out my mother had cancer, I fell apart. But because of my mother's intention to rely on God through it all, I was able to follow her lead and find my own calm, curiosity, and courage for the journey, with God's help. I hope by taking time with this book, you will find yours too.

—Judy Naegeli, Seattle 2020

PREFACE

"*PRUDENCE! PRUDENCE! TAKE CARE!*"
Our French-speaking host waved goodbye from the rustic doorway of the hiker's hut on the Mont Blanc trail. On this glorious cloudy day in the French Alps, we hiked upward for a daylong traverse to the next refuge.

At the top of the Alpine ridge two hours later, we blithely perched on boulders, eating sausage and cheese. A light mist moistened the atmosphere, but soon dark clouds enveloped us and thunder boomed overhead. Lightning struck nearby.

"We gotta get off this ridge!" my husband, Andy, shouted over the din.

We scrambled down the rocky trail, looking for safe cover. Wind gusted. Rain pelted. Thunder deafened. Lightning sliced the air.

Heart pounding, I rounded a bend in the trail and stopped dead in my tracks.

Before me was a steep, snow-covered hillside stretching downward to my right, ending in a mound of sharp talus two hundred feet below. The trail traversing this slope ahead of me was blanketed by snow of unknown depth or stability.

My feet resisted commands. My breathing stopped. Fright interpreted the danger before me. Visions of an unstable snowfield compromised by rain fueled my dread of being swept downward into skeletal wreckage on the boulders below.

Struck by fear of lightning. Terrorized by impending death. Paralyzed by panic.

Fear, terror, and paralysis—understandable reactions to imminent danger—launch a person with fight-or-flight adrenalin into the one choice she is capable of making: stand ground or run. Alarm of this magnitude serves human survival instincts well. Sometimes, abject fear is exactly what enables a person to act quickly and with physical strength. I've never scrambled over rocks with such agility as that day in the Alps.

But a chronic state of fear is unsustainable because it shuts down the brain's creativity for problem solving. Worries without resolution spin in an energy-draining eddy. Over time, if alarm devolves to ongoing anxiety, we lose hope, enjoyment, and the ability to think beyond our worrisome circumstances. Not a way to live.

I know this because I was raised in a household defined by my parents' worry and anxiety. My mother suffered the range from social discomfort to panic attacks, my dad from perfectionism to selective hoarding. They each managed their anxieties differently, with medication, a sheltered life, or rigid control of surroundings and circumstances. Their four children, of whom I was the first, were constantly warned of lurking health issues like diabetes or tooth decay. Obsessive frugality was the family's insurance against financial hardship.

While my parents unintentionally clouded our family in anxiety, our society was also dealing with its own destabilizing developments. During my impressionable childhood years, Americans feared nuclear war, communism, and cancer. Since then, circumstances have shifted. Nuclear war has been deterred by treaties and global pressure. Communism has largely been discredited as a viable political and economic system. But cancer still strikes wide-ranging fear: of getting it, of being treated for it, of dying because of it. Cancer anxiety is a thing.

So you can imagine the swirl of emotions that surrounded me when I—a healthy nonsmoker—found out I had advanced-stage lung cancer in the fall of 2013, at the age of sixty. This serious diagnosis tweaked all the sensations that could have sent me spinning. But standing in the eye of the storm, I felt a serenity that comes with accumulated trust. Life experience as a mother and pastor-teacher invited me to face this particular threat in new ways. Fighting and fleeing were not the only options. In fact, God's presence had nurtured a personal Christian faith that allowed me at this turning point to say, "Okay, Lord, whatever you desire for me. I just want to see your purposes at work."

I processed events in the six months from diagnosis to final treatment by writing a journal. My sleep pattern was altered by new routines, and I found myself awake and alert in the wee hours of the morning. So I would shuffle to my desk and ponder the previous day's activities, looking for signposts to God's presence or prodding. Scripture readings fed my soul and inspired my spiritual growth. Reflections and responses flowed into journal entries. The fruit of that daily discipline is the chronicle that follows.

Three main arcs emerge and intertwine in my story. The first is the progression of events related to my diagnosis and treatment of lung cancer. The second is the calendar, particularly as it follows the church year, which reminds me annually of God's purposes and saving actions. Remarkably, my health timeline paralleled the flow of the church year: Ordinary Time, Advent, Christmastide, Epiphany, Lent, and Easter. The third arc was subtle and its significance obvious only at the end of my tale: an evolving relationship with my mother.

This is not the book for you if you are seeking tips on how to cope with cancer, steps toward a cure, or medical advice. At the end of the book you will find patient navigation tools produced by fine cancer support groups to address those topics.

You will find this book helpful, however, if you are a patient who has come down with a life-threatening disease or developed a condition that you don't deserve, are not ready for, and feel too anxious and overwhelmed to face. My hope is that you can slow down, calm down, and get curious about what is happening to you physically and spiritually. For those of you who help patients through life-threatening disease—doctors, nurses, caregivers, even pastors—my intent is to provide emotional and spiritual resources I have summoned from forty years of pastoral experience to complement the clinical information you share with the sick.

Many of my friends were shocked by the news of my diagnosis and assumed that I was devastated. I was not. Did my emotions shut down? Did denial take over and cloud my perception of reality? Or did something else rescue me from a steep fall into terror?

I invite you to absorb my account and judge whether my story helps you find your calm center amid cancer anxiety. *Prudence!* Take care!

INTRODUCTION

Ordinary Time

FLYING HOME FROM AFRICA, I started to cough.

Early in the second leg of our journey from Nairobi, I felt a cold coming on—a normal occurrence for me during and after air travel. But before we landed at San Francisco International Airport on August 18, 2013, the sickness had already sunk into my chest—*not* normal—and within days escalated to a full-blown, constant bronchial cough.

My husband, Andy, and I had ventured to East Africa for three weeks of vacation and ministry travel, punctuating visits to Christian mission sites in Kenya and Uganda with spectacular wildlife safaris. Dancing ostriches surprised us. Lanky Maasai intrigued us. Exuberant children amused us. And devoted missionaries inspired us. We crossed the equator, the Nile, and the Kenya-Uganda border, carried by our driver, Andrew, in a robust Toyota safari van. Navigating unsigned and unpaved roads into rural areas, we met friends doing God's work among people learning business, children going to school, the sick seeking treatment, and prisoners finding justice.

Could this cough be a delayed reaction to the dust of the rural areas we had toured? Mysteriously, it did not seem to develop into pneumonia or infection. It just hung on inconveniently for weeks. Meanwhile, once home, the plan was to resume our early-morning hiking routine, pack our backpacks, and head for the Sierra Nevada on Labor Day weekend. The climax of our end-of-summer celebration was to hike to the top of

Half Dome in Yosemite National Park. I had been training for this challenge for months, acquiring the precious wilderness permit in the spring and hoping I could join the family's Half Dome Hall of Fame and cross the feat off my bucket list.

Our first Saturday home, we planned a hilly five-mile training hike around a local reservoir. My cough required taking it slow, so we brought lunch and expected a two-hour circuit of the lake.

I was shocked to be exhausted by the twenty-minute mark, gasping for air.

"Andy . . . I am having trouble . . . catching my breath."

"Andy . . . slow down . . . I can't keep up."

"Andy, I think I need to turn back."

We hadn't even scaled the first hill. Andy eyed me with concern. He could hear my wracking cough and wheezing, so that was that. We turned around and went back to the car. Doubts that a climb of Half Dome was even possible upset me all the way home.

It turned out Yosemite was just not meant to be. My chest cold persisted, and on the day of our departure, a wildfire erupted on the west side of the park. Radio news reported prodigious amounts of smoke blanketing the Half Dome area. It would be foolhardy to undergo the physical exertion of a steep mountain climb under such conditions. We dolefully lugged our backpacks out of the car and, dejected, ate rehydrated backpack food for dinner.

After six weeks of coughing and general exhaustion, I finally saw my primary care physician, Dr. Paul Endo, a gentle man and an astute diagnostician. I described my symptoms. "I just want to feel better. I can't sleep. I'm tired of coughing." Dr. Endo agreed that six weeks was long enough to suffer and, because of my history of mild asthma and bronchitis, prescribed a round of Zithromax in case a secondary infection had gotten a foothold.

Meanwhile, the fall schedule descended upon our household. Though Andy and I were empty nesters, we were not retired. Andy was an engineer who designed small medical devices, like pulse oximeters that clip on your fingertip to measure oxygen in your blood and glucose monitoring devices for people with diabetes. I was a pastor and adjunct seminary professor, dividing my time between congregational responsibilities and academic pursuits. Our calendars were always a patchwork of interesting activities and obligations reflecting our love for life. That September we enrolled in the Oakland Symphony Chorus for a musical challenge, and I started teaching a Bible study at a local church. Maintaining these commitments through the fall turned out to be increasingly difficult, however, as I continued to weaken.

The Zithromax, a strong antibiotic, fostered no improvement. After another two weeks of bronchospasms, the weight of not knowing what was going on made me pensive and unwilling to make short-term plans. I worked at home, so my schedule was flexible, but I didn't feel like doing much. With growing concern, I returned to the doctor. Dr. Endo explored the possibility of "reactive airway disease," in which a person's airways go into hyperdrive, reacting allergically to a phantom irritant. To break the cycle, he prescribed the steroid Prednisone. But just to make doubly sure I did not have pneumonia—which he could *not* hear in my lungs—he ordered a chest X-ray.

Three hours after the chest X-ray, Dr. Endo called. "Don't take the Prednisone! It looks like you might have pneumonia after all."

He prescribed another broad-spectrum antibiotic and a follow-up CT scan—standard protocol, apparently. Defeated by this news and exhausted from side effects of the new medication, I suspended my Bible study and underwent the scan three days later.

The imaging technician, young enough to be my son, greeted me and blithely pattered, "Let's see, we're looking for that mass in your left lung. Okay, let's go!"

Gulp.

Three days waiting for test results, over a weekend, seemed an eternity. At 7:30 on Monday morning, Dr. Endo called to confirm a mass in my upper left lung that required further investigation. He mentioned biopsy.

"It could still be pneumonia, but I want to get an interpretation from a lung specialist. I'm sending you to Dr. Michaela Straznicka with hope that she can get you in this week for an evaluation." An online search revealed she was a thoracic surgeon specializing in lung cancer. This felt ominous. And worse, the earliest appointment I could get was on Friday—another five days to wait.

My uncertain health, not to mention the muscle strains caused by the cough, overcame me. I found myself getting tense and anxious. Every bone in my body wanted to plan out my calendar for the next six months. Every thought in my head, however, hit a dead end of uncertainty.

Friday finally rolled around, and Andy joined me for the appointment with Dr. Straznicka. At 8:30 a.m. the cramped waiting room was already a tableau of detached, anxious humanity. CNN was playing on the flat-screen TV, mesmerizing patients until their names were called. When my turn came, we were ushered through the office maze into the examining room painted vivid red and cream, with French-inspired plaques and pictures of fanciful designer shoes. The attending nurse saw us chuckle and admitted, "Yeah, this is definitely *her* room. The other docs wouldn't be caught dead in here." Soon we heard a purposeful clacking crescendo down the hall, and a statuesque blonde in four-inch red heels greeted us with a warm smile and gravelly cheerleader voice.

Getting down to business, she described what she saw in the CT scan. She used analogies and word pictures to describe my condition and interpret the images. She talked very fast ("Sorry, I'm from Brooklyn"). This vivacious, funny woman with a very active right brain reassured us with her knowledge, her experience, her thorough explanations, and her upbeat attitude.

But the news was less upbeat. She continued, "Both the X-ray and the CT show a solid mass 5.9 centimeters by 5.1 centimeters—about the size of a racquetball—embedded with clear borders in the upper lobe of the left lung. See it here? It is nestled against the mediastinum, the center of the chest where your aorta, esophagus, and trachea are situated." Among four potential explanations, she ruled out a cyst and an abscess, leaving two possibilities: an opportunistic infection like Valley Fever, or, more likely, a cancerous tumor.

The cancer possibility prompted myriad inquiries: Is it the primary site or a secondary appearance? If the latter, where is it elsewhere? She looked closely at the CT image and couldn't find any indication that the local lymph nodes were excited or alert to the mass. When I looked at the image myself, I said, "That looks big to me." And Dr. Straz replied, "Yep, it *is* big, and it's camping out in some pretty expensive real estate."

The first task was to find out what it was, and that called for a biopsy.

She added reassuringly, "It is definitely treatable." Surgical removal was necessary no matter what it was. We set up an appointment for the lung biopsy six days hence, on Halloween, with a follow-up appointment the following Monday, November 4, to hear the report.

I fretted about what this was doing to my short-term schedule. If lung surgery was around the corner, how long would I be out of commission? It felt more and more like a life-altering situation.

The lung biopsy by bronchoscope is an outpatient procedure done in the hospital's operating room. I was wheeled in at 10:50. My eyes flickered open in post-op recovery at 1:40, and by 2:40 I was sent home, a little shaky.

The most apparent discomfort was a sore and scratchy throat, due to the breathing tube and lights-and-camera conduit sent down my windpipe. The pain I felt as the medications wore off was located where it had hurt to breathe while hiking since May! Was that how long this mass had been growing?

Despite the mounting ambiguities of my situation, during this particular medical procedure I felt secure emotionally—no fear, anxiety, or sense of abandonment by God. In fact I felt spiritually covered under the warm blanket of God's love. And to be honest, anesthesia helps one float through this experience. In one-step-at-a-time mode for now, I remained peaceful and curious about what was to happen.

Having pledged to be transparent about my health issues with daughters Katy and Judy, I talked with each of them when I got home. They both lived in Seattle, and distance prevented face-to-face reassurances we would have wanted to give each other. But thankfully the initial shock they experienced when I notified them of the lung mass earlier in the week had worn off. Now, they were upbeat and interested in medical details.

Later in the day as sedation fog dissipated, my mom, who also lived in the Seattle area, surprised me by calling to ask how things had gone. This communication was out of the ordinary—shocking really—since she had called me maybe five times in my entire adult life. Why she would call at this point can only be explained by a mother's worry. I did not know at the time that my mother would subsequently call weekly until Christmas to check on my progress. But on this day, my voice was too congested to sustain further conversation, so Andy took over and gave her the report.

That night I couldn't sleep. I began to journal my experience, thanking God for all the friend and family support I was getting: Andy's tenderness, Rogene's ministrations, Sue and Curt's soup dinner, the staff at John Muir Hospital, and my surgeon's skill. It was very reassuring. I was also reminded that God was the quality assurance officer on my case; he would keep me safe. Very skilled human beings were operating as God's agents, even if they didn't know it yet. Trusting God with the process, I waited for the pathology report, which wasn't expected until Monday. I was really beginning to hate weekends.

Over the next few days, recovery from this biopsy was much harder than I had anticipated; loss of sleep, a worsening cough producing copious amounts of phlegm, and the wait dragged me down. I felt depressed, and my body was a sob ready to burst.

Saturday was a gorgeous fall day, but I was lethargic. I felt guilty that we were not hiking or somehow taking advantage of the weather. Life had gone into slow motion, each moment weighted with an unknown lurking in mind and body, waiting to see the light of day.

As was our Saturday custom, we talked over the plan. Andy started by saying, "I'd like to turn over the vegetable garden today . . ." Typically he would follow this with "Wanna help?" But instead his voice softened. "Would you like it if I set up the hammock so you can be close to me while I work?" His acceptance of my weakness and the tenderness atypical of my fix-it engineer husband caressed my soul. His quiet appreciation of my new limitations inaugurated a season of patient attentiveness.

Andy suspended our hammock between apricot and plum trees. A gentle breeze brushed away the sun's warmth, so an afghan was added for insulation. He helped me into the swinging bed, and I nestled into its folds in perfect, restful equilibrium. Held so securely in the hammock, underneath a fluttering, filtering leaf canopy, my emotional dam burst, and I started to weep.

I am not prone to tears and had not yet cried through the weeks of discomfort, imaging, and ambiguous news. God's calming presence spoke. "I am carrying you, just as this hammock is holding you up. You are safe in my care." Pent-up anxiety surfaced and surrendered to God's peace. Resting in the grace of Jesus Christ, I prayed and absorbed the spiritual reinforcements God provided. Having silently named the possibilities of cancer and death for the first time and soaking in divine reassurances, I felt strengthened for what was to come.

This serenity was not unprecedented. Over a sixty-year lifetime, life had shaken me severely on numerous occasions. Through all of those events, God had been faithful and steadfast.

On that stormy hillside in the French Alps, Andy crossed the steeply sloped snowfield ahead of me. Despite his reassurances, my feet remained immobile. Suddenly from behind came a French-speaking man in a bright-red rain poncho, who sized up the situation immediately. "*Allez, allez! C'est sûr d'aller!* Go, go! It is safe to proceed!" He waited, giving further reassurances, but it wasn't until he began to whistle a happy tune that I felt my feet unglue from the hillside and take the first few steps into the snow. Andy's footprints guided me forward, and the Frenchman's song propelled me from behind. At the far side I thanked our new friend, who disappeared around the bend and was gone. To this day, I believe he was an angel of God.

God has a good track record in my life, and the challenges have stretched my faith, made me more durable, and given me confidence that nothing can truly overwhelm me. This much was settled: no matter what "this" turned out to be, I had every reason to believe that God would accompany me and keep me safe in his arms.

ADVENT

1 🌿

A "Come to Jesus" Moment

Thursday, October 24, 2013

As a pastor, I have attended countless parishioners through illnesses and hospitalizations. Part of my responsibility in those situations is to be a non-anxious presence and empathetic listener. Calm and empathy are hard to fake. I have discovered that the deeper my spiritual life, the more authentic and transparent I can be. Now that I am the one facing a life-threatening illness, that same spiritual grounding provides the rock beneath my feet even when it feels like the earth is moving.

Learning how to remain calm and empathetic has been my lifelong project, since anxiety riddled the home of my upbringing. In retrospect, knowing firsthand what world-class worrying looks like has been a gift to my ministry. But at the time I left home, I had no idea how much my life had been burdened by fear and anxiety, trained into me by my mother. As a young adult, I identified anxiety by name, and knowing intimately its corrosive potential in the spirit, I was motivated to overcome my inherited propensities. Over decades I have been released from knee-jerk reactions to the unknown, the unexpected, the challenging, and the painful. This relief has emerged slowly through demanding pastoral duties and teachable moments. Ultimately, the emotional freedom I generally experience now is the fruit, I believe, of a direct healing work of Jesus Christ in my life. I have come a long way and I am grateful.

But today I am beginning to feel a burden. This developing medical situation hangs over me like a cloud. My instinct is to research, ask questions, do *something* proactive to relieve the tension building up. I've made all the appointments, and several tests have been ordered. I can do nothing now but wait for things to unfold. I hate this.

My thoughts go a mile a minute in the middle of the night. Full of questions, bereft of answers, I feel the weight of uncertainty about what is going to happen. I want to say, "This isn't like me; I should just get over it." But it *is* like me.

Responsibilities beckon. Meetings, events, and organizational work await my attention. Today I am supposed to participate in a conference call to strategize with colleagues around the country. Locally I am consulting with a church experiencing conflict. This work ordinarily stimulates me, and everyday challenges summon my best efforts.

What I am finding, however, is that busyness-as-therapy is not working for me. My mind drifts, I cannot concentrate, I get antsy. It feels like my primary calling has shifted from church work to medical navigation, with no map and no clear destination other than "perfect health" to guide me. Where do I go with this?

A wonderful hymn, "Come, Ye Disconsolate," issues the invitation:

> Come, ye disconsolate, where'er ye languish,
>> Come to the mercy seat, fervently kneel.
> Here bring your wounded hearts, here tell your anguish;
>> Earth has no sorrow that heav'n cannot heal.

The mercy seat is Christ's throne, the very center of God's heart. Jesus is the one who can do something, particularly when we feel exhausted and powerless.

> Come to me, all you who are weary and burdened, and I will give you rest. Take my yoke upon you and learn from me, for I am gentle and humble in heart, and you will find rest for your souls. For my yoke is easy and my burden is light. (Matthew 11:28–30, NIV)

Stepping back for perspective, I realize I have been given the gift of slow motion, a chance to settle down spiritually. I have an opportunity to work out my feelings and actively trust God with my life. If Christ's claim is true, I am going to find out how Jesus is *my* non-anxious presence and empathetic listener. He says, "C'mon, I know you've got all this unresolved stuff to handle, but I can help you rest in the midst of it. Let me guide you. Don't worry; I will be gentle and tender with your spirit. You'll see!"

And that is where I must leave this, trusting Jesus to keep my burden light. Where else could I go?

2 &

Assigned to the Waiting Room

Friday, November 1, 2013

How do we deal with the reality that we have been assigned to the waiting room?

My friend, Janice, herself a breast cancer survivor, gave me a timely word of encouragement. She knows firsthand how hard it is to be assigned to the waiting room. Take me to the ER! Take me to physical therapy! Take me anywhere the issue can be resolved, please! But the waiting room? Bleh.

While waiting for my hair appointment on Wednesday, my attention strayed to the guilty pleasures offered by the stack of magazines. Reading them took me out of waiting mode and into diversion mode. One way to cope with the waiting room is to say, "Let's do something completely different, something we don't have to wait for, while we're waiting for this other thing to happen." Doing something that offers immediate gratification is a common way of coping with the interminable.

What else can we do while waiting? We can simply stop doing anything. Twenty years ago I lived in Zimbabwe for four months while on sabbatical from my pastorate. I remember waiting with hundreds of others in thirty- to forty-minute lines at the post office in Harare, Zimbabwe. Waiting is a fact of Zimbabwean life. On any given day, fifteen lines of at least thirty people each would wait to pay school fees or telephone bills and to buy stamps. Not a single person other than myself (after learning the first time) had brought a book to read or drums to play or other family members with whom to converse. The blank stares revealed a deep sense of hopeless resignation.

When our precious Plan A has been thwarted, we look for distractions or go into a holding pattern. We are tempted to divert our attention from Plan A to something else or to do nothing out of depression or a sense of futility. We often feel that until we arrive at our ultimate goal, we can't get anything else done. That is *exactly* how I feel right now, awaiting diagnosis.

Through the prophet Jeremiah, God addressed this waiting game with the dispirited Jews of the exile upon their arrival in Babylon (Jer. 29:4–9). They were saying, "How can we [possibly] sing the Lord's song in a foreign land?" (Ps. 137:1–4). God said, "I have a plan; there is a better way to handle your exile!" Similarly, the apostle Paul exhorted the church of Thessalonica to balance its anticipation of Christ's second coming with the challenges and calling of the present, to evangelize and to engage in productive labor.

These Scriptures invite me to look at the waiting room in a different light. Could it be that rather than waiting *for*, the better way involves waiting *on*? The prophet Isaiah conveyed this promise to the people: "They that wait upon the Lord will renew their strength" (Isa. 40:31 KJV). In Hebrew, the word translated "wait" means "wait in focused anticipation."

God declares that we will find strength by waiting on the Lord. A period of forced inactivity or rest is disquieting to an athlete who is itchy to get back to daily workouts. But forced rest is also the opportunity to strengthen the mind, the motivation, and the mettle for future competition. My baseball hero, Giants catcher Buster Posey, was out for one year with a severe ankle injury. He returned to help San Francisco win the World Series in 2012. Was he ready? You bet! But only because that entire year on the disabled list was programmed to help him regain his strength and stoke the fire in his belly.

In the same way, those of us on an equivalent disabled list have the opportunity to gather our resources and inner strength for the moment when the gates are lifted and the King of Glory beckons us forward again.

But what do I mean by "waiting on the Lord"? I've found it helpful to observe a good wait staff at a local restaurant. Fine waiters focus their attention on the customer and have learned to read nonverbal signals of satisfaction or need. The really good ones don't even have to ask, "Is everything all right here?" or "Do you need anything more?" They just *know* and unobtrusively minister the dinner graces that make a meal memorable.

What would it look like for me, a person in a medical holding pattern, to wait on God? To wait in focused anticipation in this context means remaining alert to God's desires, ready to do his bidding at the table set before me. It means actively cultivating intimacy with the Savior and renewing a commitment to follow in Christ's footsteps. It means taking the time to review my beliefs and covenant commitments and to revive life skills. It means keeping an eye on what God is looking at, never losing sight of the people around me who need Jesus, and standing ready to respond to their spiritual, emotional, and physical needs.

During Hitler's rise to power, much of pastor Dietrich Bonhoeffer's frustration was directed at his own church, which was so enamored of the chancellor that it capitulated doctrinally. Bonhoeffer, seeing the official Lutheran Church compromise its core beliefs in order to remain legitimate in the state's eyes, kept his focus on training new pastors. His way of waiting on God was to form a secret seminary, invest in the lives of future preachers, and respond to the faulty theology that was undermining the church's witness. Even imprisoned, his writing kept him focused on the main thing and left for us a grand legacy of spiritual reading.

The test of my own effectiveness at waiting on the Lord is my readiness, when the time is complete, to move forward in strength and conviction. In a way I feel I have been waiting for seven years, since I left my last pastorate, but only if I think in terms of waiting *for*: waiting for a new pastoral call, waiting for a stable teaching contract, waiting for my first grandchild. But all along, moved by circumstances into a quiet lifestyle, God has been strengthening me inwardly. And though I might not have been aware of it during those seven years, the spiritual workout this represents has prepared me for whatever is to come, even this week. No matter what direction the Lord wants to propel me, I am assured—as one who has been waiting on the Lord—that all will be well, and I will be ready.

3 ✣

The Diagnosis

MONDAY, NOVEMBER 4, 2013

THE THORACIC SURGEON STRODE INTO her red examining room with the pathology report in hand. Andy and I wondered how this conversation was going to start, but she, who has delivered this news many times before, just said it: "Well, Mary, it is cancer."

In retrospect I am amazed that I did not panic or even get upset. Andy was with me, and the skills I learned through marriage to an engineer kicked in: listen, take notes, ask questions.

"The biopsy took a lot longer than usual. I had a pathologist in the operating room looking at samples to make sure I had gotten something usable. It took fifteen tries before I found live cells to send to the lab."

Dr. Straznicka continued. "So here's what we found: the tumor is a squamous cell carcinoma, a non-small-cell cancer. At least three lymph nodes are also positive, which bumps us up to Stage III."

We asked questions, looked at the CT scan pictures again, and discussed next steps.

"Some imaging needs to be done to see if the cancer is anywhere else, so a PET scan and a brain MRI should be done right away. I've already made an appointment for you with Dr. Gigi Chen, an oncologist, who will talk over the treatment options."

Because the tumor is nestled against the central structures (aorta,

trachea, and esophagus), it is inoperable now. The goal is to shrink it—
we hope in the right direction—to create the necessary margin.

It is a bewildering new world, and as the surgeon said, "You're going
to be busy for the next few months."

The news shocks me for several reasons: 1) This type of lung cancer
is found primarily in people who have smoked, which I never have; 2) I
have virtually no family history of cancer and no obvious risk factors; and
3) I just turned sixty, in perfect health. This ball has come out of left field.
I'm still getting my glove on to catch it. The first thing Andy said as we
left the surgeon's office was, "So much for clean living."

Nobody in my family dies of prolonged illness. My father died suddenly of a cerebral hemorrhage; both sets of grandparents died of heart
attack or stroke. Andy and I have had no experience caring for family
members over any length of time. Will my family take care of me? Do
they know how? I guess God has appointed me the object of a teachable
moment for us all, because one thing I know for sure: I'm committed to
months—if not years—of messing with a life-threatening disease, and
I'm going to need some help to get through it.

4

Awaiting the Redemption of Our Bodies

TUESDAY, NOVEMBER 5, 2013

ONE WAY I COPE WITH difficulties is to ponder and write. My best time for this is early in the morning before the world awakes. By contrast, in the evening, pondering turns to fixating, which turns to obsessing, and nothing good comes of that. It is far better at bedtime to offer a prayer of submission and commit my problems to the Lord.

But in the morning, we are down to business, God and I. I not only can see the facts simplified but also gain insight. With a clear head, the great assurances of our Savior and shepherd are a hug to my soul and a spur in my side. Out of that place of serenity and resolve, I can then sort out my emotions, God's thoughts as revealed in the Word, and possible responses to the day's events and challenges.

Difficulties and testing are in my future. In this refining moment, I must relate my very real Christian faith to the very real dangers of this life and determine how I shall *be*. I believe it is in my power to choose how to think, how to feel, and how to act under these circumstances.

And so, with the news that I am now contending with lung cancer, I am inspired by one of the greatest chapters in the entire Bible, Romans 8, starting at verse 18:

> I consider that the sufferings of this present time are not
> worth comparing with the glory about to be revealed to us.

> For the creation waits with eager longing for the revealing of
> the children of God. . . . For in hope we were saved. Now
> hope that is seen is not hope. For who hopes for what is seen?
> But if we hope for what we do not see, we wait for it with
> patience.

Yes, I am groaning and waiting. But I am not afraid, and I am not
devastated by this news. I pray that—through the process God has appointed me to undergo—I will be calm, curious, and courageous. I believe God is working out his purposes for my redemption and resurrection behind the scenes. I can't explain it, but I possess hope and feel
perfectly safe. It is not a curriculum I would have chosen—"this year I
am going to become an expert on lung cancer"—but the teacher in me
is going to become a student of the medicine *and* of the Great Physician.

5 🍃

My Life under Scrutiny or The Folly of Denial

WEDNESDAY, NOVEMBER 6, 2013, 6:30 A.M.

Today every inch of my body will be scanned, a PET scan first (neck downward), then a brain MRI (head only), checking to see if the cancer Beast has gotten out of its cage. I am groping for images to describe this growth inside my body, and I find myself reverting to the graphic depiction of evil found in the book of Revelation: the beast. Ironically, those cancer cells that have multiplied and gathered in my chest are *my* cells gone awry. Out of control, they have become a new, foreign, and hostile entity, much like the computer, Hal, in *2001: A Space Odyssey*. It wants to take over my body, but if we can discover how far it has roamed, we can grab hold of its tail and slay it. The first step in that discovery process is medical scanning.

I welcome the scrutiny as a necessary step to my cure. Without that specific knowledge of the disease's progress, the Beast cannot be slain. Gone are any pretenses of privacy or the sovereignty of my own opinion. I mean, really, what good would it do for me to say, "Y'all, my insides are none of your business. There's nothing wrong with me, and I can take care of this cough on my own. C'mon, if we all *say* there's nothing wrong with my lungs, there *isn't* anything wrong with my lungs." Folly, right? And completely self-defeating.

While undergoing this medical scrutiny, I am prodded to ask how I feel about the spiritual scrutiny to which I am subject as a beloved child of God. Jesus said, "It is not the healthy who need a doctor, but the sick; I have not come to call the righteous but sinners" (Mark 2:17). What he meant was, as long as I claim I am spiritually well, I am not going to find any help from him. But once I recognize my need for God, I will be met and treated by the Great Physician. What is my ailment? In the body my sickness is labeled "cancer." In my spirit the fatal spiritual illness is sin (Rom. 6:23), and we were all born with it. Unless we acknowledge our symptoms, submit to the scrutiny of God's examination, accept the diagnosis, and take the medicine, we will die of it.

And yet, just look at the spiritual gymnastics we perform to avoid acknowledgment of wrongdoing and submission to discipline, such as: No, I'm not really sick . . . well, okay, I've got a little food addiction going here, but it's not hurting anyone. Or, I was born this way (a compulsive liar, a glutton, a worrier), and therefore my behavior should be celebrated as authentic, the "real me."

Well, it may be the real me, but *I* am seriously deluded if I do not see the danger of my condition. It is only a deeply rooted case of pride that fuels such a delusion. That is precisely the spiritual problem for which God offers the spiritual solution.

So what do we do about this wrong-headed self-determination? We turn ourselves in. We chime in with the psalmist's plea: "Search me, O God, and know my heart; test me and know my thoughts. See if there is any wicked way in me, and lead me in the way everlasting" (Ps. 139:23–24).

We confront in our heart of hearts the reality that nothing is hidden from God. His motive for making known our true state is a desire to see our healing and redemption. We are wasting precious time as long as we insist that we have nothing to be healed of. If we can get over this spiritual hurdle, "the way everlasting" opens to us and a new life is possible. This is the life Jesus promised in his teaching, secured by his sacrifice on the cross and delivered through his resurrection from the dead. It is ours; all we have to do is acknowledge our sickness to get the help that is freely given by our Savior.

But can you believe it? We even need God's help to get up the gumption to be scanned for sin. This is the point where the Holy Spirit makes the reminder call, checks our spirit to verify we know the way to the doctor, and then takes us there.

> Likewise the Spirit helps us in our weakness; for we do not know how to pray as we ought, but that very Spirit intercedes with sighs too deep for words. And God, who searches the heart, knows what is the mind of the Spirit, because the Spirit intercedes for the saints according to the will of God. (Rom. 8:26–27)

What kind of Christian would I be if I stood down from my defiant denials of sin and instead let God begin the deep work of transformation? I know the answer to this question because in the year before I gave my life to Jesus Christ, I was conceited and self-righteous, believing myself to be a completely fine "Christian" because I went through all the appropriate motions others could see. But what was happening internally, at the prodding of the Holy Spirit, was a gentle invitation to submit to God's spiritual diagnosis and to let God reign in my soul. What relief I felt in the act of acknowledging my helplessness against sin and my dependence on the Savior to break free. As a humble and contrite member of God's family, I can accept the defeat of spiritual cancer eroding my soul, even as my medical helpers seek to overwhelm the cancer that has taken root in my lung.

Thanks be to God for putting me through the test.

6

Tests and Images

TODAY I MET WITH MY new best friends, oncologist Dr. Qi Qi (Gigi) Chen and radiation oncologist Dr. Sophia Rahman.

Dr. Chen possesses petite stature, a quiet and gentle manner, and slightly accented speech. Her active listening and warm giggle are accompanied by a razor-sharp intelligence and prodigious memory. She becomes my primary care physician for the duration of my treatment, specifically focusing on the ongoing effects of chemotherapy.

Dr. Rahman is a striking brunette with compassionate brown eyes and a sweet, almost daughterly, manner. Honestly, this oncology practice oozes grace. Dr. Rahman's part will be to design and deliver what may be the more difficult of the two treatments. She articulated the reasons for radiation and presented some scary consent forms.

Each of these women spent forty-five minutes with me to debrief my situation and explain the proposed treatments, based on what they observed in yesterday's scans.

Here's what I learned:

My lung cancer is Stage III-A, determined by the size of the tumor—that is, larger than 5 centimeters—and the involvement of three lymph nodes, one across the midline. The PET scan and MRI gave a clearer picture of the extent of the cancer, which has a tendency to metastasize to bone and brain.

Here is the good news: The cancer has not migrated beyond the observed lymph nodes.

The cancer will be overpowered and defeated—we hope—by six weeks of daily radiation and concurrent cycles of chemotherapy, starting no later than November 18. This treatment plan will render me feeling lousy by the end of December, I am told. At that point, the team will evaluate my progress with more imaging, and the surgeon will determine if resection (removal of the lung lobe) is possible.

What a remarkable learning opportunity this is. How good God is to attend me and show his kindness in little ways throughout this day. The MRI, which many dread as claustrophobic and noisy, was actually fun. The rhythms and tones of that clacking machine reminded me of some joyous moments in Uganda this summer, as well as some exhilarating concerts at the symphony.

On tomorrow's agenda: surgical implantation of a Vein Access Port to facilitate delivery of chemotherapy—one more fasting day in anticipation of a surgical procedure.

7 🍃

On Assignment: A New Perspective
on "Call"

THE CHRISTIAN CHURCH OFTEN USES the term "discerning one's call" to refer to the process of figuring out one's vocation. In my tradition, the Presbyterian/Reformed stream of the church, that call is sensed and validated in community. My personal call, exercised as a pastor-teacher, has shaped my identity and brought structure to my life since 1987.

The last seven years without a full-time pastoral position in a congregation has stretched me. The quiet life that has evolved has enabled me to write, to counsel, to earn a doctoral degree, to fill pastoral gaps as they occur, and otherwise to serve in quiet, thinking ways. Nevertheless, I have felt like I was waiting for something to happen.

And then cancer strikes. Could this be that "something"?

While I am still getting used to saying "lung cancer" out loud, life has taken a sharp turn into an entirely new world. My medical vocabulary is expanding daily. My new best friends are oncologists, dosimetrists, technicians, phlebotomists, nurses, and front-desk receptionists. My days are now scheduled with medical consultations and imaging appointments. Today I go under anesthesia once again to have a chemo port installed in my chest. It's all extraordinary activity I have never ever had to do myself, though I have walked alongside many people before me who have taken this journey.

The temptation is to cry out, "When can we get back to a normal life, Lord? When can I return to work? Lord, this is such an interruption—I can't get anything done! I am not able to do the ministry you set out for me! I'm supposed to be teaching and ministering the sacrament." Yada, yada, yada.

And God says, "Huh? You are most certainly doing the ministry I have laid out for you. I have sent you on a new assignment." Jarring thoughts of Jonah come to mind . . . Moses . . . the apostle Paul . . . Mary. All reassigned to participate in God's great purposes.

I've been trying this idea on for size for the last few days, and it's sticking. I realize my call has always been the Lord's assignment, not my pursuit. Just like a buck private in the army, I am subject to the will of my commanding officer. When God says, "Go," I go; when God says, "Go there instead of here," that's what I am to do. So I have been reassigned duty to the waiting rooms, examining rooms, procedure rooms, and laboratories of the medical establishment. And already I am finding ministry opportunities *just by sitting there*, because my new best friends are also needy men and women looking for hope in this world.

A few weeks ago I was in the waiting room of a breast cancer center in Oakland while my second mammogram that week was being processed. A few of us ladies were in our fluffy white spa robes waiting our turn when one of the women turned to me and said, "I think I've met you before." I didn't recognize her, but when she started telling her story, I remembered where our paths had crossed. We had the most amazing conversation, in which we shared the anxieties of mammography and past false positives.

I realized God had put me there to minister to this woman.

My follow-up mammogram came back perfectly clear. Was that second trip to Oakland a waste of valuable time? No way! On God's assignment I was right where he wanted me to be, to offer companionship and reassurance, white robe and all.

Whatever skills we have developed as gospel ambassadors, whatever strength has enlarged our hearts, whatever experience has pierced our soul or lifted our countenance . . . these are all transferable assets in God's marvelous economy.

For the time being, my office is my recliner; my mission field comprises the various rooms where I am getting stuck, imaged, instructed, or medicated; but my *calling* is God's assignment, which he can redirect at any moment. I proceed with the apostle Paul's awareness proclaimed in Romans 8:28: "And we know that in all things God works for the good of those who love him, who have been called according to his purpose."

The great lung adventure is not a detour. It is taking me right into the middle of God's claim and call on my life. I am beginning to rejoice in that truth.

8 ✒

Paring Down to Nothing

Friday, November 8, 2013, 7 a.m.

YOU MIGHT APPRECIATE THE BOND between a woman and her purse. If not, it's like this: Don't mess with me, baby. My Baggallini bag has provisions for body, mind, and spirit in the form of water bottle, protein bar, mini New Testament, wallet, sunglasses, inhaler, lipstick, last week's church bulletin, iPhone, pencils and pens, cough drops, car keys, iPad, and lip balm. And that's just the beginning. At any given time I have everything I need to spend most of the day away from home.

But the lung cancer adventure requires a new ritual. Almost daily this week, in preparation for one procedure or another, before leaving home I must divest myself of my purse ("all valuables") and most things on me: earrings, cross pendant necklace, watch, rings, sunglasses, and extraneous clothing. As I arrive at the medical office/surgicenter/hospital, the only items stashed in my cargo pants are my driver's license, health insurance card, a credit card for the copay, and my phone. Once I go through that door, though, even those items are relinquished, as well as my own clothes, in exchange for the blue-and-white hospital gown (a funny name for such an inelegant garment). And they keep asking if I am hiding anything else they want: dentures, contact lenses, or hearing aids.

So what do you do with yourself, in a strange environment, with lots of time on your hands, nothing to read, and no props to make you feel at home?

Earlier this week I panicked because I had left a John Grisham novel on the kitchen table by mistake. But thankfully God grabbed me by the scruff of the neck with a big smile and said, "Oh good, let's just sit together and make our own fun." Immediately the thirst in my soul quickened, and for once I was grateful for the quiet and freedom to talk things over with my Great Physician. The ongoing conversation required a bit of confession and forgiveness too because, frankly, I'm tired of paring down to nothing.

Maybe that's why Jesus sent the disciples out to minister in towns and villages with these instructions: "Take no gold, or silver, or copper in your belts, no bag for your journey, or two tunics, or sandals, or a staff" (Matt. 10:9). He wanted to make sure their faith was placed firmly in Jesus and their dependence upon the Lord was a real, tangible trust.

Jesus hopes we might discover that a person doesn't need that much stuff. Too much gets cumbersome, causes its own worries, and closes us off to the relational security available to us. Solid faith requires no outward props or provisions to flourish when we sit with our Savior and enjoy life together.

When we come to church toting our cell phones, a latte, and maybe some crocheting for the back row, we are actually coming to worship empty-handed spiritually. Securing ourselves against boredom or hunger in fact dulls our senses to our spiritual need and the excitement of God's presence in worship.

If we were to come to the Table without travel insurance or security blanket, we would discover our hands and hearts are free to grasp the love of God without hindrance and in full trust for his provision. "What then are we to say about these things? If God is for us, who is against us? He who did not withhold his own Son, but gave him up for all of us, will he not with him also give us everything else?" (Rom. 8:31–32).

The answer is, "Yes, he will!" God has given everything of his own so that we would have everything we need from his hand. So I am leaving my hands free for a while to be ready to grab God's hand for stability and receive from him all I need.

9 ☙

I Got a Tattoo!

Friday, November 8, 2013, 3 p.m.

Today's rather mundane pretreatment preparations included a trip to the cancer center for another CT scan. My radiation oncologist and a dosimetrist are designing a radiation strategy that finds the safest pathways for those six radiation beams to enter my body, converging on the tumor. The radiation techs also fashioned a cradle to position my body for each radiation treatment. They applied three tiny tattoos—specks that will be lined up with the laser beams to ensure that the tumor is accurately targeted. I have a mental picture of the Death Star blowing up in *Star Wars*.

My assignment during the next week is to practice shallow breathing so that when I am in the radiation machine, I can stay very still.

10 ✑

The Downside of Playing It by the Numbers

Monday, November 11, 2013, 4 a.m.

I HAVE LIVED WITH MY diagnosis of lung cancer for just one week now, though I was strongly suspicious for a week or two prior to that—enough time to start getting my head and heart around the possibilities. During that period, many sleepless hours—induced by my cough and an antibiotic—provided ample opportunity to satisfy my curiosity on the World Wide Web. I wanted to educate myself about lung cancer but discovered instead a tree of bitter fruit. One number made me pucker in dismay—the average five-year survival rate of 17 percent.

Averting my eyes from the screen, I made a decision: I'm not going to do this by the numbers. I am not going to obsess on this statistic or that probability. Call it denial if you want, but I choose to fix my eyes on the One who knows my future and who is going to nurture me toward it. I choose to take one step at a time and make sound decisions for my health and healing, without fear of the odds. Why use my precious energy spinning in hopelessness when I can thrive in God's energizing love?

So many Scriptures come to mind, one sent this morning by a long-time friend:

My [child], pay attention to what I say;
> listen closely to my words.
Do not let them out of your sight,
> keep them within your heart,
for they are life to those who find them
> and health to one's whole body.
(Prov. 4:20–22 NIV)

Instead of feeding myself disheartening statistics, I will nourish both body and soul by steeping in God's Word. It reminds me of God's power to redeem and heal, Jesus's love that carries us, and the Holy Spirit's ability to do what is humanly impossible.

Jesus only got exasperated with his disciples when they could not grasp how imminent and available was God's help. In Mark 6:35–44 Jesus and the twelve have rowed across the Lake of Galilee to a quiet place for a meal and some rest, only to find the crowds have arrived first. Jesus sees how thirsty they are for the kingdom of God, so once again he preaches almost all day. By five o'clock everybody is tired and hungry, and the disciples, going by the numbers, are distressed that so many needy people out there in the boonies might cause a riot.

Jesus says, "No, no, let's see what we have available right here in our midst." The disciples find a little boy with a lunch big enough for himself—five loaves and two little fish—but ridiculously inadequate for a crowd.

The disciples say, "No way, Jesus. This isn't going to be enough."

But (I imagine) the Lord says, "This is plenty! Go and organize the folks into eating groups, and I will get the food ready." Then Jesus thanks his heavenly Father for what he has been given and asks the disciples to feed the people with it. The distribution begins, and there is an abundance of food for everybody—thousands of people—with leftovers too!

There's only one number in that story that is important: One. The One and only, Jesus the Lord, is able to do the very thing that is needed. No odds, no probabilities, no statistics to consider, except the certainty that God "is able to accomplish abundantly far more than all we can ask or imagine" (Eph. 3:20).

Too many of us play it by the numbers. Defining success by how much we have, how high our income is, how many vacations we take, how expensive the car we drive is, how high the SAT scores our kids achieve, or how sharply we dress diverts our attention from the One whose love for us cannot be measured. Our success scale is a human invention. God places infinite value on loving us. His complete love drives away anxiety about any other measure of our worth.

It is not playing it by the numbers that guarantees our well-being, but sticking close to Jesus. Faith in the one who gives life and health according to God's Word will bear fruit we can't even imagine. "What then are we to say about these things? If God is for us, who is against us? He who did not withhold his own Son, but gave him up for all of us, will he not with him also give us everything else?" (Rom. 8:31–32).

11 ✣

The Treatment Plan

Today was another long, tiring day, but I obtained plenty of good information to satisfy my curiosity:

- The full-body PET scan and brain MRI from Wednesday showed no further spread of the cancer, beyond the tumor and the known lymph nodes.
- The PET scan did indicate that my "bone marrow is working very hard." The oncologist said she is quite confident there is no cancer in the bone marrow, but it is excited about something, perhaps increased inflammation. To investigate further, . . .
- Tomorrow I will have a bone marrow biopsy, done in-office with a local anesthetic, if for no other reason than to have a "before" picture in advance of the chemo onslaught.
- Wednesday will be the dress rehearsal for my radiation treatment, when all the players sign off on the plan.
- Thursday, radiation begins and will be conducted every weekday morning at 8:40 for six weeks. It is a brief procedure, efficiently conducted. On nonchemo days, I will be home by 9:20 a.m.
- Monday, November 18, chemotherapy begins on a four-week cycle: One full week on, three weeks off. Repeat as often as necessary, but typical of cases like mine is a four-round course of treatment.

The chemotherapy consists of Cisplatin (on Mondays) and Etoposide (Monday–Friday), plus a cocktail of antinausea medications. Cisplatin and Etoposide are old standby chemo drugs, in use for almost thirty years, and have proven to be very effective with my kind of cancer.

The chemo counselor met with me this morning to go through all the side effects and how they are treated. I would love to be one of those patients for whom the side effects are no big deal. But the biggies are nausea, gastrointestinal disturbance, hair loss by the end of third week, and immunity suppression. No Christmas parties for me this year.

I have a half-inch stack of papers to read on all this stuff. What an education!

God is still good, and God is still strong.

12 🍃

The Supportive Community

THE DAYS PREPARING FOR MY cancer treatments have been amazingly busy. Because my protocol involves both radiation and chemotherapy, my medical team conducts two tracks of testing and preparation. Today I go in for a dress rehearsal of my custom-designed radiation treatment to ensure the high-energy X-rays will converge on the Beast. Yesterday it was a bone-marrow biopsy to set a baseline for measuring side effects of chemotherapy.

Another kind of preparation is happening at home. Because the disease itself has already made me feel sick and tired, it is apparent that I will need help for the duration. And so, using a task-coordination website called Lotsa Helping Hands, friends are signing up to take me to and from treatment, stay with me afterward until Andy gets home from work, and bring meals. It is heartwarming and moving; the volunteers represent members of three churches I have served, old friends, current students, and even my daughters' pals.

Truly, "it takes a village" to heal a person. Quite often gospel accounts of healing involve a third party requesting Jesus's help for someone who is sick.

One of the best illustrations features the four friends who worked to get a paralyzed man to the feet of Jesus (Mark 2:1–12). The crowds were so thick around the Teacher/Healer that the four friends got creative.

Since they couldn't get in the front door, they devised a plan B. They climbed onto the roof and somehow got the supine guy up there, too, and started pulling away at the roof tiles to gain entry from above. Just picture the resourcefulness, patience, and determination of these friends. A bit of harrumphing went on inside, I imagine: Who is going to pay for the damage to the roof? But Jesus was very impressed with the friends' faith and persistence and addressed the sick man directly. Their plan worked. The man was healed spiritually and physically right before their eyes.

Four friends gathered around me last night to pray for my healing. Their tenderness, persistence in prayer, and faith in the power of God lifted me up. The prayer warriors of our church are alert and interceding for me; other saints throughout the country and even around the world are carrying my family and me to the throne of grace. I find great comfort in this dynamic and trust that God has heard the cries of his people and will act according to his purposes for me, the church, and the kingdom of God. What a great feeling!

13 ✍

This Is Going to Hurt

Thursday, November 14, 2013, 4 a.m.

ONE OF MY ALL-TIME FAVORITE movies is *Hook*, starring Robin Williams, Dustin Hoffman, Julia Roberts, and Maggie Smith. There's this great scene where Captain Hook (Hoffman) is stealing the affections of the kidnapped children of grown-up Peter Pan (Williams). Hook is making more progress with the already alienated son, Jack, than the younger daughter, Maggie. Soon we see Jack dressed up as a miniature Captain Hook, but one thing more is needed to complete the costume: a pierced ear to accommodate a big gold earring. As the captain holds up his arm hook, the tool of choice for ear piercing, he gleefully utters in Jack's ear, "This is *really* going to hurt."

On Tuesday the nurse practitioner didn't say it quite like Hook, but she warned me that my bone-marrow biopsy would hurt at a certain stage, principally because I have very strong and hard bones. She was right, if only for a minute or two.

Aside from the additional evidence that I am going into this adventure generally healthy and strong, her warning points to a dynamic we have been taught to welcome in the Christian life: It is going to hurt in the short term, but later it will be okay. Various Scriptures come to mind: "I consider that the sufferings of this present time are not worth comparing with the glory about to be revealed to us" (Rom. 8:18); "Weeping may linger for the night, but joy comes with the morning" (Ps. 30:5b);

and "Jesus began to show his disciples that he must go to Jerusalem and undergo great suffering . . . and be killed, and *(oh, by the way)* on the third day be raised" (Matt. 16:21). And my personal favorite: "Discipline always seems painful rather than pleasant at the time, but later it yields the peaceful fruit of righteousness to those who have been trained by it" (Heb. 12:11).

It helps to know that a little investment in a painful discipline now will yield something good in the end. I am hoping the result of my treatment is freedom from cancer for the remainder of my earthly life. Getting there is going to be a rough go, and God is making me strong for the challenge. But even if that is not the outcome in store for me, I am assured our sovereign Lord has blessings already flowing into my life, his abiding presence will sustain me, and godly peace will surpass my understanding. Some of these can only be experienced through a period of painful trial, but God is the glorious victor:

> Who will separate us from the love of Christ? Will hardship, or distress, or persecution, or famine, or nakedness, or peril, or sword? . . . No, in all these things we are more than conquerors through him who loved us. For I am convinced that neither death, nor life, nor angels, nor rulers, nor things present, nor things to come, nor powers, nor height, nor depth, nor anything else in all creation, will be able to separate us from the love of God in Christ Jesus our Lord. (Rom. 8:35–39)

14 🌿

First Radiation Treatment

Thursday, November 14, 2013, 8:15 a.m.

THE TALLY FOR THE LAST seven days: one IV, two blood draws, two shots of local anesthesia, one biopsy needle, and three mini tattoos. Now I understand why people describe this part of the cancer experience as "pin cushion."

Besides that I have a dentist appointment late this morning to fill a cavity discovered on Tuesday. Add one, maybe two, Novocain shots to the total.

I am off to my first radiation appointment. I have been briefed, prepped, practiced on, and otherwise ushered through the process, so during the procedure I expect no anxiety.

This morning I arrive early, having allowed too much time for commuter traffic, but they take me right in. I have my own cubby, supplied with this week's gown. You go to the dressing room, change, and get ushered past "the bridge" and into the treatment room.

The lead-lined room where the high intensity X-rays are delivered reminds me of the engine room on *Star Trek*. You stretch out on a table, around which imaging machines and the X-ray emitter rotate on cue.

Once I'm lying down in my custom-made upper-body cradle, my job is to relax and remain still. I am highly motivated *not* to wiggle; it's not hard and is, in fact, a relaxing way to begin the day. No strange noises, nothing weird about it. I spend the time in prayer and thanksgiving for all the resources gathered to help me. And then it's over, in fifteen minutes.

Afterward the tech rubs my upper back with a calming lotion to stave off potential sunburn. Since they are ahead of schedule, the techs offer to let me see the big machine. A drum of high-tech mechanisms, lights, and moving parts, at least five feet in diameter, rotates behind the wall at the head of the patient's cradle. It really does look like *Star Trek*! The techs describe enthusiastically what this linear accelerator does and how it is tailor made to my body's structure. Before the invention of computers and atom smashers, none of this was possible.

15

Resting in Uselessness

During treatment on my first day of radiation, two realizations blessed and entertained me:

First, the awareness of my utter uselessness in the present moment and the all-surpassing power of God. Last week my inner CEO came out as I prepared for battle engagement. I cope with stress by getting organized and managing the challenge as a project.

But in the large radiation room, my sole job is to lie down on the table, put my arms over my head, allow the technicians to position me exactly in line with the lasers, and then remain still for fifteen minutes. That's it. No reading, no iPod, no talking—just remain still and take regular, shallow breaths so my tumor doesn't move beyond the tolerances built into the program.

Meanwhile, some of the most astounding healing technology imaginable is at work around me. Out of the wall behind my head come three arms carrying imaging devices and the high-energy X-ray emitter, the head of the gantry. These arms are almost noiseless—inaudible when they are actually engaged in their work—and operated by remote control from the bridge. The arms rotate above, below, and around me and deliver the radiation to their target. Behind the wall is the body of the linear accelerator that powers their concentrated beam into the Beast within my chest.

My job is to be still and rest. I can't even breathe deeply in order to relax. Something far greater has to put me in that place of relinquishing all control. That one, of course, is our almighty and merciful God. "Be still, and know that I am God! I am exalted among the nations, I am exalted in the earth" (Ps. 46:10).

Second, the idea that the energy helping me during treatment is available because God, who holds all things together, created it. I am comforted knowing the Healer created tools that righteous people can use for good.

My imagination worked backward from the photons to their source. I really don't know the science, but at some point the power of light is unleashed for healing good. Those gamma rays were endowed with energy—pent-up, disciplined power. Their "life" was created by God who, as pure spirit from the very beginning, was the only source of energy. For the good of all creation, God harnessed that power into light, atomic energy, and an orderly world. One can use that energy for bombs or for healing; I, for one, am glad for the healing.

For those in the midst of a busy or noisy life, resting in God is a stretch. How often are we secluded in a room, alone, silent, and useless? We actually try to avoid this. Radiation is teaching me that when God is present, a boisterous, joyful activity is working behind the scenes to heal and make whole. I can stand down and accept that, or I can wrestle with God and impede his work. Jacob tried that (Gen. 32) and ended up with a limp. So I have chosen to use this "useless" quiet time to remember Scripture verses I have memorized, to enjoy the humor of my supine helplessness, and receive the healing that God is effecting in the whole process.

> [Jesus says,] Come to me, all you that are weary and are carrying heavy burdens, and I will give you rest. Take my yoke upon you, and learn from me; for I am gentle and humble in heart, and you will find rest for your souls. For my yoke is easy, and my burden is light. (Matt. 11:28–30)

Yes, we have a yoke and a burden, but the load is somehow lifted and shared by the one who lugged the cross to Golgotha, who bore our sins and carried our sorrows. I am counting on that as I carry this cancer burden. We are so accustomed, in twenty-first-century American culture, to making things happen, to being useful and even powerful. Today I choose to be still and acknowledge God: the one with power that surpasses my imagination and who contends, with precision, with the Beast I face.

John Fisher, in his 1974 album *Still Life*, sings a lovely, simple song, "Rest in Him." This has been running through my head all day:

> Rest, rest in him,
> Your work is through.
> Lean back on his great power.
> He'll work through you.[1]

16 🌿

Bone Marrow Report

SATURDAY, NOVEMBER 16, 2013

PRELIMINARY RESULTS OF MY BONE-MARROW biopsy came in yesterday afternoon: no evidence of cancer in the bone marrow. This news was expected but reassuring, nonetheless. My cancer stage remains III-A.

More specific testing has been ordered to determine the cause of the proliferation of white cells. Last year's annual physical showed all blood counts were normal. Something has developed since then; my white count is triple what is expected.

Is the phenomenon related to fighting cancer-related inflammation or to some other preexisting condition? If related to the cancer, then of course we treat the cancer and kill the Beast. White count should eventually settle at normal levels. If something different is causing it, we keep a close eye on the white count to see how it behaves and act accordingly. In both cases, we proceed with the treatment plan and start chemo on Monday. Having a few extra white blood cells in the bank when initiating a process that suppresses the immune system is not a bad thing.

It's a beautiful day, and Andy and I celebrated life by going out for crab benedict, a real treat. In anticipation of losing my ability to taste, I've indulged in favorite foods this week: sushi, French food, homemade beef stew, and pumpkin spice latte.

17 ✑

Slaying the Beast

Four weeks ago today my doctor told me there was a mass in my upper left lung. Two weeks ago it was identified as a cancerous tumor. In the effort to get my head around this new reality, I have occasionally referred to this tumor as "the Beast" and have written in terms of slaying it. I am unaccustomed to mythical battle language. Nevertheless, the image sticks in my mind because there is a foundation of truth underneath it.

Unlike Don Quixote, whose imagination led him to believe he was being attacked by giants, I am not tilting at windmills. I am indeed fighting something that does not belong in my body. This intruder gained entrance by some silent mechanism, and I have resigned myself to the mystery of its origin. But its reality aligns with the spiritual battle in which all Christians are each engaged, whether we realize it or not.

The gospels depict Jesus contending with evil spirits that were wrecking lives. It was believed that demons caused various maladies: seizures, mental illness, crippling, and blindness to name a few. When Jesus cast out the demons, the illnesses disappeared. The physical and spiritual problems are linked. I hasten to add that observing a link does not fully explain the suffering we face. I do not intend to claim that whatever we endure is only a spiritual problem. But I believe the New Testament teaches that we are integrated human beings, whose spiritual lives affect our physical condition, whose psychology affects our spiritual lives, and whose physical condition can distress both our minds and our spirits. No problem is exclusively physical or psychological or spiritual. To eliminate the possibility that we may be seeing trouble in all three areas is to deny the full arsenal of tools and weapons God has given us. When we must address a health issue, we are also called, at the very least, to attend to the spiritual aspect of it, while seeking relief through medicine or psychotherapy as needed.

Engaging imagery to describe my enemy, the Beast that prowls about my chest seeking cells to devour, has been helpful. In 1 Peter 5:8, Peter uses this apt metaphor to describe the Evil One. He refers to a roaring lion, which was a considerable foe in his time and place, as it would be in ours.

Just like cancer cells, which go into hyperdrive to reproduce and take over healthy structures, Satan attempts to satisfy its insatiable appetite by attacking vulnerable human beings and destroying them. It is a perversion of God's good creation for previously healthy cells to multiply furiously and turn upon their host in order to wreak destruction. As a person whose theology starts in the perfect garden [of Eden] (Gen. 1–2), I find this perversion outrageous. It is why I consider cancer an enemy, a Beast that must be slain.

The physical battle must be fought. I am approaching it as a test of mettle and a sharing in Christ's sufferings. If I may more dearly appreciate the suffering Christ endured as a human being who died on the cross for me, even physical pain and discomfort can bring about spiritual healing. This does not stop me from petitioning God daily to slay this Beast and save me from the side effects of chemo and radiation. But if by use of chemo I can be healed of this cancer, then I gladly walk the road that so many others have already trekked.

Compared to the glorious might of our Lord and Savior, this spiritual enemy is small, impotent, and deluded. It cannot stand and survive an encounter with the living God. It boasts far more power than it actually has, but it knows that "a single word may fell it." From a spiritual standpoint, this Beast is doomed.

In the meantime, Jesus is bearing the load and carrying me through treatment. All of this is a sign to me that someday Jesus will reign victorious over *all* creation!

18 ✍

First Chemotherapy Treatment

Monday, November 18, 2013, 5:30 p.m.

Day 1 of chemo delivery went very well today, notable for all the good things:

- A Vein Access Port that worked great and painlessly. There will be no need to put IV lines in my arm or hand veins.
- A comfortable recliner with an attached table—nice! On future days I can bring reading and sewing projects.
- A window view of resplendent fall color outside.
- Shorter duration than I expected, only four and a half hours.
- Discovery that companions are welcome. Andy sat with me for an hour until he felt it was okay to go to work, but not before bringing me a great deli sandwich for lunch.
- All systems go; that is, proof of healthy, responsive kidneys. No joke intended here—Cisplatin can be hard on the kidneys, and every effort is made to flush the toxic chemo out.
- Church friend Rita's cheerful face and ride home afterward.

Today was also a good experience for all the things that did *not* happen:

- No nausea at all. The nurse identified one of the IV bags as "the Mercedes of all antinausea medications." I believe her.

- I didn't even get sleepy, so yes, I will need to bring activities to pass the time. Today I had with me the *NY Times* crossword, my iPhone, a journal/notebook, my DayTimer, and a John Grisham novel. Tomorrow I might take my quilting handwork, now that I know the danger I will barf all over it is minimal.
- So far so good in the taste buds department.
- And the best of all: I have stopped coughing! Now *that's* a side effect I will welcome!

Only one little pause today . . .

During the administration of Etoposide, I began to feel flushed and sweaty. Not dizzy, not faint, just really warm and drippy. After I confirmed this was *not* a menopausal hot flash, my mere mention had three nurses consulting, checking blood pressure (120/61, after arriving this morning at 150/74) and other vitals. No fever, no other symptoms; but because it was quirky, they stopped the infusion for twenty minutes, then resumed. I continued to feel warm, but nothing else was off. The sensation did not come back with the Cisplatin, for which they *do* expect side effects every once in a while. The experience improved from then on.

Tomorrow we'll see if the same thing happens. It may just be my normal, and I can certainly live with that.

19 ✑

Thinking outside the Chemo Cubicle

TUESDAY, NOVEMBER 19, 2013

YESTERDAY WAS MY FIRST DAY of the full treatment protocol: radiation at 8:40 a.m., and a lengthy chemotherapy infusion starting at 9:15 a.m. Surprisingly, it was a very good day.

When I arrived at the chemo dispensing area, a large open-plan room divided into maybe fifteen cubicles like a Dilbert-style office, the place was quiet. I was the first patient. My assigned space faced a window of fall color that filtered soothing light. Nurse Judi explained each step of today's treatment and got my infusion started efficiently but with a warm responsiveness that would carry throughout the day.

As the hours passed, the activity level in the center increased. Most infusions were much shorter than my six-hour stint, so a river of humanity flowed in and out of the place. Everyone announced their arrivals to the nurses by the required "full name and date of birth," so I became aware of a gentleman age ninety-one across the way.

The most intriguing patient, however, was the forty-five-year-old woman who moved in next door. She brought a friend (who sounded like an entourage), and the two conversed nonstop throughout the morning. A third unidentified voice would chime in occasionally. They discussed upcoming Thanksgiving plans, conversations over cocktails, gossip concerning their community, and other care plans related to the patient's illness. They also discussed religious and spiritual topics. I heard someone reading from Romans 8 and something about a son-in-law who was an atheist—no, an agnostic—what's the difference? they asked—and references to churches they had attended, including one I had served for ten years as a pastor.

Forget about the needle in my chemo port, forget about my confinement—it was torture not to be able to stand up, lean over the cubby wall, and enter into this conversation with my new neighbor. I thought about it, but I couldn't get past the confession, "Um, I've been eavesdropping on your chitchat . . ."

So I didn't say a word.

As I awake early this morning and replay this scene, everything I have read and absorbed about being a Christian embedded in the world comes flooding joyfully into my soul, reminding me again of the change in my duty assignment and God's call in my life. I don't feel guilty about refraining from sharing the gospel with a neighbor. I am convicted about the difficulty of getting out of our Christian cubicles and entering into the conversations going on in our neighborhoods.

Could we—could I—be so focused week to week on feeling better spiritually that we forget we are recipients of a comfort to be shared? "Praise be to the God and Father of our Lord Jesus Christ, the Father of compassion and the God of all comfort, who comforts us in all our troubles, so that we can comfort those in any trouble with the comfort we ourselves have received from God" (2 Cor. 1:3–4).

Our neighborhoods, workplaces, and coffee shops are beckoning us to share the life of Christ in authentic encounter. Eventually we will have to hang out and enter the conversations that are happening around us.

I *am* stuck in an actual, comfortable cubicle this week, but most people are not. Can we get a little curious about what people around us are talking about? Do we detect any experiences or circumstances we have in common? Has God given us a love for our neighbors? Since I am indisposed at the moment, would you go in my stead to build a bridge between Jesus and one lost soul? Just tell them "Mary sent me"—assuming it's still hard to say, "Jesus sent me," though that is the more accurate statement. It's time to "think outside the chemo cubicle."

20 🍃

Side Effects Balancing Act

O N DAY TWO OF CHEMO, all is well in my little chemo cube—not even the protracted "hot flash" of yesterday. The antinausea drugs cause constipation; the chemo drugs tend to cause diarrhea. So I am experiencing some mild gastrointestinal distress this afternoon; I have instructed my gut to fight it out.

I fall asleep when I get home, which seems normal for a nice fall afternoon. I am relieved by the cessation of my cough. The nurse I told was delighted and said it's possible the tumor is shrinking already, due to the attack upon it from all sides.

My appetite is good, and food tastes normal so far. I feel so grateful for the prayers of my friends, which I believe are being answered, and for the food they are bringing each night because I am too exhausted to cook.

21 ✑

To Live Is Christ, To Die Is Gain!

THURSDAY, NOVEMBER 21, 2013

THE NEWS OF THE REV. Dr. Henry Greene's death silenced me this week. My dear friend and colleague in church renewal work died suddenly on Monday, doing what he loved, hiking in Yosemite National Park. Henry was the real deal, a genuine-to-the-core Christian who lived for Christ in all he did.

As a result of his sudden passing, I am thinking about death from a different perspective. Believe it or not, my diagnosis of lung cancer just seventeen days ago did not evoke such thoughts of my own demise. I have avoided living by numbers and statistics and have chosen to put my trust in the One and only. But today I must think about death, not only Henry's, but my own.

To guide my thoughts, I turn to a passage of Scripture in which the apostle Paul, imprisoned and writing back to one of the churches he served, pondered his fate.

> [I hope] that by my speaking with all boldness, Christ will be exalted now as always in my body, whether by life or by death. For to me, living is Christ and dying is gain. If I am to live in the flesh, that means fruitful labor for me; and I do not know which I prefer. I am hard pressed between the two: my desire is to depart and be with Christ, for that is far

better; but to remain in the flesh is more necessary for you.
(Phil. 1:20–24)

It is Paul's joyful affirmation that speaks to me, confined as I am to my recliner: "For to me, living is Christ and dying is gain." Henry is experiencing now the "dying as gain." He is embraced by our gracious God, without a wrinkle on his face, with a pure and restored heart, without a care in the world, completely enraptured by the beauty and glory of God. He has gained everything for which he lived: reconciliation with God and restoration of his soul in the grace and mercy of God's forgiveness in Jesus Christ. Whatever burdens he was carrying—and I assume, as with most pastors, his were heavy—have now been lifted from his shoulders. Whatever sorrows he bore have been transferred to the crucified Christ permanently, and he is laughing with that deep voice we all grew to love and look forward to. Henry has peace with God.

I, on the other hand, have the chance to live in my earthly body a while longer. Left behind, I nevertheless cling to the same spiritual blessings Henry has received: reconciliation, peace, burden-free trust in Jesus, and every spiritual blessing available in Christ. I say clinging because most of the time this is faith, pure and simple: the evidence of things hoped for without seeing them as Henry now sees them. But they are mine, just the same. For me, "living is Christ" means I have the deep and joyful privilege of making Christ known through trusting and demonstrating his love and forgiveness in my new world of cancer treatment.

By the time Paul wrote the letter to the Philippians, he was living under a threat of death. But we must clarify that death itself was not a threat to Paul at all; it was the threshold into new life. That is why he could say he could take it either way, live or die. The only thing he didn't want was to dishonor Christ; his heart was focused only on exalting Christ's name. Nevertheless, the choice was a hard one, and Paul would prefer to die and see Christ face to face. But for the time, as with me, Paul realized his duty assignment as proclaimer of the mysteries of God's will was still in force.

This is how I feel about my own life at the moment. Jealous as I might be about the way Henry spent his last day and was transferred into eternity, God has a different plan for me. I see even more clearly that my call is to continue to encourage people of faith, to equip them for their duty assignments, and to rejoice in *their* successes along the gospel way.

When I heard the news about Henry, my immediate thought was, *What a way to go, bro!* The expedience of God's call upon his life was breathtaking. But in the next instant, I said, "No! Too soon, too soon!" That word came out of the selfish side of me that relied on Henry's ministry in my life and in the wider church. But Henry leaves behind a cadre of church members, loving family, and colleagues and friends who resolve to complete the earthly tasks we have been assigned. And so we shall persevere in joy and faith, knowing "to live is Christ."

22 ✐

A VAP and the Flow of the Spirit

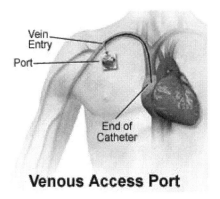

Vein Entry
Port
End of Catheter

Venous Access Port

Two weeks ago I had a Vein Access Port (VAP)[2] surgically installed just below my left front shoulder. Its purpose is to provide reliable access to a central vein for the infusion of chemotherapy. A little drum

---

[2] Illustration by Bruce Blaus—Blausen.com staff (2014). "Medical gallery of Blausen Medical 2014." WikiJournal of Medicine 1 (2). DOI:10.15347/wjm/2014.010. ISSN 2002-4436. Accessed at https://en.wikipedia.org/wiki/File:Venous_Access_Port_Catheter.png. Used with permission under Creative Commons License, accessed at https://commons.wikimedia.org/wiki/User:BruceBlaus

was embedded completely under the skin and a catheter threaded into the vein above the heart. At each chemo session, the nurse punctures the drum with an IV needle that delivers the medicine. This method minimizes infection and saves veins in the arms and hands, which are not always the most comfortable sites for such an intrusion.

You can imagine how important it is to keep my VAP channel clear. At the end of each drug infusion, the VAP is flushed with saline and a bit of Heparin (a blood thinner) to prevent clotting and future problems. A clogged VAP prevents the proper exchange of fluids necessary to get me well: blood draws for testing as well as intravenous infusion of various drugs.

Once again, my imagination carries me to the sort of infusion that is very much a part of the Christian life: the inflow and outflow of the Spirit of God.

First, the inflow: The God of the universe dwells in and enjoys the beauty and bounty of all he has created. He resides in eternal and unlimited grace, power, blessing, and provision. God has never needed anything: he has always had enough time (eternity), knowledge (omniscience), power (omnipotence), and self-sustenance (provision) to get along. I love how Christian philosopher Dallas Willard described him: "God leads a very interesting life, full of joy. The abundance of his love and generosity is inseparable from his infinite joy. . . All of the good and beautiful things from which *we occasionally drink tiny droplets* of soul-exhilarating joy, God continuously experiences in fullness!"[3]

This joy and beauty and the experience of heaven simply cannot stay there—it overflows into our experience. God cannot contain himself! God's limitless resources (including love and comfort) spill over into all creation, flowing through Jesus Christ to and into each one of us. "God's goodness and generosity is lavished upon us, whom he loves!" (Eph. 1:6). This is the inflow of the Holy Spirit: "God's love has been poured into our hearts through the Holy Spirit that has been given to us" (Rom. 5:5).

In fact, God could paralyze us with the sheer force and power of his bounty. In wisdom and understanding, he dispenses his grace in doses

---

[3] Dallas Willard, *The Divine Conspiracy: Rediscovering Our Hidden Life in God* (San Francisco: HarperSanFrancisco, 1998), 62f, emphasis added.

we can handle to meet our ongoing need and store some extra grace for when reinforcements are required.

Then, the outflow: God expects the blessings he has lavished upon us to overflow into the lives of others. The abundance of God's provision assures there is enough blessing for us to share. We can clog the lines, so to speak, by hoarding what we mistakenly think is scarce and failing to expand God's benevolence beyond our own narcissistic sphere. Stuck in a limited view of what God *wants to do through us* is often enough to stop the flow of the Spirit's gifts and power.

Because we do clog the line with attitudes inconsistent with the reality of God's spiritual blessing, we need a flushing out through confession and a declaration of God's forgiveness. As we are used by God to dispense his love and care to others, we must also submit to his cleansing, keeping the channels open by avoiding a puny faith or hoarding instinct.

Today I am rejoicing that, despite my growing fatigue and need to sleep, God pours out enough blessing to pass along to nurses, fellow patients, and companions. I pray that more of us might discover the vast reservoir available and that we would have the courage and faith to welcome more than a mere trickle of God's infinite blessing.

23

The Best Dinner Ever

FRIDAY, NOVEMBER 22, 2013

IT'S FRIDAY, AND I'VE HAD seven radiation treatments and five chemo infusions in the last nine days. Although yesterday was my most fatigued day, I am still doing well. Today I went with the flow and slept all afternoon. After dinner I watched a wonderful movie with Andy and even stayed alert through the whole thing.

It was indeed a very good day, in the company of Matt, my morning driver; Anne, my chemo nurse; Jane, my afternoon companion and hydration enforcer; and of course Andy, who got home early on a Friday night. Phone conversations with my daughter, Judy, and spiritual director, Floyd, filled in a lovely day of God's blessings. Friend Karen brought the perfect dinner for our table tonight, and on day five of chemo I could taste every morsel.

Two weekend days off from the rigors, then back in the chemo cube and radiation tunnel on Monday.

Good news of a medical nature: Dr. Chen says the blood marrow studies are done, and all is well. White blood cells are reacting with appropriate vigor to the onslaught of foreign terrorists and should settle down soon, once the Beast begins dying. No other cause for the elevated white count can be identified. My blood pressure is 118/70, my other blood work is strong, I have had no nausea or other unpleasant GI effects, and a very encouraging medical workup this morning makes me feel like this thing is doable.

24 ✑

Taste and See That the Lord Is Good!

I HAVE OFTEN SAID THAT God's biggest competition in my life was food. Of the seven deadly sins, gluttony has been at the top of my personal list too many times. So you can imagine how I anticipate the possibility of losing taste while undergoing chemotherapy with Cisplatin. Any medicine with the word "platinum" in the name can't be good for a foodie like me.

I have been wondering when this taste bud transformation would take place, because it hasn't yet on day nine of treatment. Tonight I celebrated that fact by enjoying the perfect dinner a friend brought to our table: roasted pork loin with baked pear slices, dilled carrots, mashed potatoes, spinach/strawberry salad, and chocolate chip cookies.

First of all, it was a Naegeli kind of meal: full of color, nutrition, fresh vegetables and fruit, lovely seasoning—the perfect dinner. But it was the cookies that did me in: homemade, fresh-baked chocolate chip cookies with walnuts and butter. I bit into that aromatic biscuit and tasted every element of it bursting in my mouth. And I just cried; it was so delicious and *good*. That one cookie may very well be the highlight of my whole Thanksgiving week.

Isn't it intriguing that the psalmist would exclaim, "O taste and see that the LORD is good!" (Ps. 34:8), and "How sweet are your words to my taste, sweeter than honey to my mouth!" (Ps. 119:103). Taste is perhaps the overlooked sense, after sight, hearing, touch, and smell. The senses are our God-given means of taking in reality—gathering what is out there and bringing it into our own experience in here. One or more of our senses may be compromised by illness or disability or enhanced by gifting; but we have a total of five to keep us in touch with what is outside ourselves. I think of autistic Temple Grandin, who organizes her world visually; blind Ken Medema, who captures and communicates his world through music; deaf, blind, and mute Helen Keller, who was finally reached at the water spigot through touch; and my three siblings and me enticed by the smell of Nana's fresh pears on an Illinois summer's afternoon. I think of Jesus, who gathered the miraculous power of God at a wedding in Cana, during which he changed water into wine that became the finest-tasting vintage of the day (John 2).

In the colorless, dim, and disorganized world of this age, the Evil One seeks to diminish our senses and prevent us from discovering God. To counteract this brazen effort, the Christian community must feature the vibrant beauty around us, thereby giving witness to the Creator through the arts. Together we can gaze at a painting by Makoto Fujimura and bleed with God's compassion. Together we can sing and make melody in our hearts to the Lord and get in touch with the grandeur of heaven like the choirs of Revelation. Together in Christian community, we can practice hospitality as one way to share the aroma and taste of God's good provision; and when we hug one another at "the passing of the peace" during worship, we afford one another the touch of God. Through all of these sensory channels the spiritual reality of God passes from God's realm into our hearts.

Let us consider what there is to taste and see of God. On Christ the King Sunday, how can we experience God as victor over the beasts that seek to work us woe? In what way can we take in the life of Christ and allow him to overshadow our fears, our discomforts, our deficits, even our disbelief? I am reminded by that chocolate chip cookie that God can break through at the most unexpected moments and shout, "I'm here! See me! Touch me! Hear me! Smell me! Taste me!" A sensory experience becomes not an end in itself but an invitation to worship the Creator and Sustainer of life. We practice this dynamic when we celebrate the Lord's Supper. When Jesus commanded his disciples to "Take, eat, this is my body given for you," and "Drink this cup in remembrance of me," he was inviting us to ingest his very presence. Jesus so wants us to appreciate that God's sovereignty in the universe is a reality in our souls.

25 🍂

Working Out the Kinks

MONDAY, NOVEMBER 25, 2013

THIS PAST WEEKEND ANDY AND I took an easy walk on Saturday morning and then hunkered down for the Big Game between Stanford and Cal Berkeley. My previously finely tuned gut is reeling with the antinausea meds. So my project over Saturday and Sunday was to find the right balance of food, water, and medicine to deal with what is now severe constipation.

I went to church but was shocked to hit a wall before the service was over. We took a seat in the back row, didn't interact with anyone or even stand up. Thirty minutes in, I was finished. Came home and slept for two hours.

I am praying for wisdom to modulate my activity as we prepare for the arrival of two daughters and a son-in-law for the Thanksgiving weekend. My home helpers are going to have some fun jobs this week.

26 ✑

Dreams of Healing

AFTER A WEEKEND OF DISCOMFORT and fatigue, I've had two very positive days and am feeling much better. Yesterday was my last chemotherapy of round one, so I have a rest from those particular rigors until December 16. Daily radiation keeps up the attack on the Beast. It should just give up now.

I had quite a night, though—profuse sweating at times, vivid dreams, no sickness whatsoever, and actually pretty darn good sleep, despite all the activity. The medical explanation for the night sweats is probably that super-duper steroid they give me with the chemo. I am subject to prolonged flushes: a red face and lots of perspiration, sometimes for hours. In the midst of all that, I had a crazy, wonderful, cast-of-thousands dream. The night sweats were draining away the cancer, every tumor, node, microscopic cell, and nefarious manifestation. I felt completely whole and unimpeded by fatigue or sickness, energized for today. I dreamed that God did this with a broad sweep of his hand and that it was a game changer, the gateway to a transformed life and ministry.

From a clinical view and what I understand about dreams, at the very least, this tells me that even my subconscious is ready to receive the miracle of healing. I am all in—body, mind, and spirit: a willing participant in treatment, a willing recipient of prayers for healing, and a willing observer of progress.

So what is healing all about? And how is it different from cure? Doctors are cautious about declaring a particular case of cancer "cured." They used to refer to "remission" and now prefer "No Evidence of Disease" (NED). As my friend, Craig Pynn, who has gone this road before me, states in a recent note: "The medical-industrial complex of cancer care cannot in good faith declare a cure, because it evaluates the situation by a different set of numbers. But just because a person may never be cured does not mean she won't be definitively healed. Healing is such a rich, multidimensional word because it encompasses the physical, emotional, and spiritual components of a whole person in Jesus Christ."

As the sign above a Christian hospital in Kenya says, "We treat, and God heals!" But there is ample evidence that God can *cure*.

Jesus cured the people he touched. We have no example of him not curing, being unable to cure, or refusing to cure. Rather, we have delightful examples of his offering cure beyond what was requested. The paralytic lowered through the roof to Jesus's feet desperately sought the healing of his disability. Jesus first cured his soul—"Your sins are forgiven"—and then, to back up the claim that he had the authority to cure the *whole* person, he said, "Time to stand up and walk!" (Matthew 9, with parallels). I doubt that chap thought much about the possibility of a recurrence, though we know that someday in his future he did die of *something*. So was he healed? Yes. Was he cured? Yes. Did he eventually die? Yes. And so it is with us.

I am absolutely assured that God is and will be healing me. I feel I have turned a corner overnight. My days are rich relationally, emotionally, mentally, and even physically, I have much to be thankful for. Will God cure me of cancer? This I cannot predict, nor do I feel that I deserve it. But I believe God is able to vanquish this puny but obnoxious foe with a stroke of his hand. Period. I do not consider my dream to be predictive of the future but descriptive of my mindset on the matter. My full conscious and subconscious are focused on God's doing whatever wondrous thing God chooses to do for as long as God desires to do it.

Another facet to the dream invigorates me: as a result of the healing I experienced, my ministry assignment was redirected, reenergized, empowered, and organized by that same healing God. I laughed and clapped in delight as God's new plan for me unfolded. A joyful season of collab-orative ministry that benefits many people is ahead. God does not want me to forget that a blessing of healing comes with a commission to be a blessing to others.

27 &

Recalibrating My Self-Sufficiency

WEDNESDAY, NOVEMBER 27, 2013,
THE DAY BEFORE THANKSGIVING

TUESDAY WAS A GOOD DAY—RADIATION ONLY, with my typically help-ful and chipper team first thing in the morning. My friend, Donna, picked me up later for the drive to Danville to get my hair cut "short and cute," as salon master Michael said. Since Friday, when the nurse practitioner said, "Everybody's different—you might not lose your hair," I have considered getting a wash-and-wear cut. I have better uses for my finite strength than styling. So that was done, and it was a nice lift.

New discomfort in my esophagus kept me up a few hours overnight. Heartburn, acid indigestion—ha! As soon as that phrase came to me, I remembered good ol' Alka Seltzer. It worked. At 5:00 a.m. I blissfully fell asleep in my recliner.

Andy, later, finding my side of the bed empty, padded downstairs to check on me. He was unhappy that I did not wake him and ask for help. "I'm an engineer! I fix things! I could have saved you hours of suffering!" His frustration flared, and I witnessed how powerless he feels as an intimate observer of his wife's cancer. So I am recalibrating my self-sufficiency once again and receiving anew the blessing of a concerned and attentive husband.

A straightforward day today; our son-in-law flew safely home from Beirut to Seattle last night. Judy, Katy, and Doug are driving eight hundred miles to join us for Thanksgiving. Let the feasting begin!

28 🍃

Thanksgiving!

THURSDAY, NOVEMBER 28, 2013

I AM THANKING GOD TODAY that all my GI and esophagus discomforts have abated and are under control. The "magic elixir" the doctor gave me coats the gullet and relieves pain. The holiday challenge is going to be pacing my eating—small bites, slow consumption, patient swallowing. But I can still *taste*! And I can still *smell*! And I still have an *appetite*!

Our daughters and son-in-law arrived at 9:00 p.m. last night, after driving the eight hundred miles from Seattle in one day. Now a lively, convivial atmosphere pervades our home, music playing, pies baking, joggers stretching for a morning run; it is truly a delight. I sit in my chair, watching and listening and enjoying.

29 ✐

Essential Identity

THE SOCIAL SITUATIONS OF THANKSGIVING week and daily conversations with my helpers have prompted reflection on how I see myself. The question is, What is my essential identity in light of what has been happening lately?

Phrases such as "my friend with cancer," "she's a fellow cancer victim," and other designations that define me (or others) by an ailment bother me a bit. I appreciate anew one of the sensitivities my husband has demonstrated for years. As staff scientist for a medical devices company, Andy designs products destined to help people who have diabetes manage their disease effectively. You notice I said "people who have diabetes" instead of "diabetics." Identifying people by a chronic disease or condition diminishes them; in reality, something far more fundamental characterizes them—their unique and essential identity. As a medical inventor, Andy provides tools that help people—schoolteachers, truck drivers, business managers, community activists, moms, dads, or children—live their lives defined by far more powerful realities than diabetes.

Or cancer.

And by the way, no one has used this term in reference to me, but just so we're clear, I am not a "victim" of cancer or of anything.

But what or who am I?

The question is an important one for Christians who have placed their full faith and trust in Jesus Christ. As a Presbyterian and Calvinist, I tend to vacillate between a triumphalist designation—"the Elect"—and a woe-is-me mantle—"totally depraved." Among Christians of all stripes, the most common identities in contention are "child of God" and "sinner." Do these labels help us or hurt us?

Some might find "sinner" a discouraging label. Are we really defined by our fallen nature before God? Is this an essential part of our character—to be flawed and sinful, weighted down by confused motives and ungodly behavior? From a biblical standpoint, the apostle Paul's essential identity as a sinner only grew stronger as he aged and became more acquainted with his own spiritual struggle. In his earlier letters he refers to himself as "least among the saints" (Eph. 3:8), but by the time he writes the pastorals, he is "chief among sinners" (1 Tim. 1:15). It was he who declared, "All have sinned and fall short of the glory of God" (Rom. 3:23). So yes, we are sinners. This is our reality and we cannot escape its truth, even now.

But when we say we are sinners, in Christ a huge "and" follows: "And [we] are justified freely by [God's] grace through *the redemption* that came by Christ Jesus." We are not only sinners, we are redeemed. That means that by God's action on our behalf, we have been lifted out of the deadendedness of sin and into a hopeful and restored life, made new in Christ. This too is our reality: "But to all who received him [the Word], who believed in his name, he gave power to become children of God" (John 1:12). So yes, we are children of God. This is also our reality, and we cannot escape its truth either.

The designation "sick" is like the identifier "sinner." It represents a reality but points to a path toward restoration: the sinner is redeemed by the Savior, the sick is healed by the Physician. You can't experience salvation without the recognition of your sinfulness, just as you can't experience healing without first acknowledging that you are sick.

So when I say, "I have lung cancer," I am admitting I am sick and in need of healing. But I do not refer to myself as a cancer victim, because a) nothing about this situation ultimately threatens my identity; b) God is moving mightily to heal me, and I gratefully receive the help; and c) my illness has not changed essentially who I am. One of my visitors this week even thrilled me by saying so: "Mary, I am so happy to see that you are fully yourself." And so I shall be, in Christ—wife and mother, teacher, quilter, blogger, mentor to the next generation of pastors, and a redeemed sinner and a child of God, who is contending for the moment with a Beast.

30 🌿

Thanksgiving Chronicles

FRIDAY, NOVEMBER 29, 2013

THANKSGIVING UNFOLDED IN A WONDERFUL way. My daughters insisted I rest and let them cook up a storm to create a lovely and complete Thanksgiving menu. But I wasn't a total blob; I dispatched *some* responsibilities within my abilities—supervising the grilling of our butterflied turkey (Andy and Judy did the heavy lifting), assembling simple appetizers, grinding the cranberry-orange relish, and making gravy, which seems to be the only kitchen skill I have not yet successfully passed along.

I ate a bit of everything—everything!—with no ill effects. A big answered prayer!

31 ✒

Thanksgiving Chronicles:
The Physical and Relational Dance

SATURDAY, NOVEMBER 30, 2013

THE HIGHLIGHT OF THE DAY after Thanksgiving was gathering the five of us for a family portrait. Photographer Tim brought his gear over and situated us on/around a teak bench in the backyard for many, many shots of this goofy family.

We devoted the rest of the weekend to the launch of Advent—Christmas activities, done mostly by others under my supervision (really, my enjoyment). The girls will get a tree this morning and string the lights, with a promise from me that whatever they do will be perfect!

All my precious family members are modulating their energy levels around me, helping me calibrate my need for rest. When things get exciting, I tend to join in without thinking and then crash or cough a lot. So I'm trying to keep an even keel. I know this isn't selfish; being awake and available when I really do need to show up requires disciplined rest.

In a departure from my very strong family tradition of going Christmas shopping the day after Thanksgiving (not the frenzied bargain-hunting; just relaxed early-morning browsing and soaking in the atmosphere), I stayed home yesterday and thoroughly enjoyed the quiet. Everybody else took off midmorning for a run or kayak around Lafayette Reservoir, and I took the opportunity to get some sewing done—even sat outside in the backyard to do so. Lovely weather and a refrigerator full of leftovers made the simple life rejuvenating.

This is all part of the physical and relational dance of which I am a part these days.

32 🖋

Finding the Well

THE TWO DAUGHTERS AND SON-IN-LAW have now returned safely to their homes in Seattle. We had a fantastic four-and-a-half-day Thanksgiving weekend. Lots of good-natured chaos, meaningful conversations, family activities, picture taking, movies, food, of course, and messes everywhere. Yes, the perfect family get-together.

I discovered it is harder to be fully aware of one's physical condition with all that noise, activity, and distraction. I found myself on occasion ready to crash, having missed the warning signals that would have gotten me back in my recliner for a rest. No harm done, but not in line with my instructions to "listen to your body" and act accordingly.

The experience reminds me, however, of a youth director with whom I worked decades ago, who crashed and burned within an inch of his life. Twice. It is not only ministers—my main circle of friends—who know how this goes. Anybody immersed in American culture can get swept into the end-of-year whirlwind. Life is busy enough, but add to it a holiday social calendar, and the pressure is on. One year Andy and I dressed up for *eleven* church-related parties in four weeks. Special events require extra effort to pull off, relational needs often intensify, expectations rise, the cookie brigade makes too many stops at the office. Pretty soon we are hanging by a thread, missing daily time with the Lord, caught up in the noise, activity, and distraction of life. Under these conditions, it becomes very difficult to listen to Jesus and act accordingly.

The quiet life God has allowed me to live the last few years has prepared me for the current challenge, I realize. When one works alone at home Monday through Friday and the phone rarely rings, one can connect thoughts and build strength for coming onslaughts. The goal of solitude and silence is not the silence itself, nor is it escape, but the serenity that comes from being in touch with the presence of God. I am quite sure that sustained periods exploring the reaches of my introversion have contributed to my non-anxious state now. My work-a-day friends and colleagues, however, are engaged in highly social and interactive environments. Can they find that same serenity and quiet with God?

In *The Desert in the City*,[4] a contemporary "desert father," Carlo Carretto, addresses the plight of city folk who do not and cannot live in a desert cave away from the world. Carretto gently advises a person on how to carry the desert within and retreat there whenever necessary to hear the still small voice of God. One initially finds that place by taking a personal retreat and meeting God in the stillness, long enough to establish its "location" and the sound of God's voice. Spiritual discipline is the practice of staying close to the well of living water and enjoying communion with God amid the desert of noise and activity.

We may not characterize our lives as a city or a desert, but wisdom dictates we recognize those dynamics in the life we have chosen. Thanksgiving weekend's buzz gave me the opportunity to practice the spiritual discipline of holy detachment promoted by the Desert Fathers. Doing so allowed me to stay in touch with my body, hear and commune with Jesus, and act accordingly as his disciple. The Lord can help us learn to glide through this season, joyfully connected to our Savior, drinking from his well.

33 ✐

The Great Cloud of Witnesses

WEDNESDAY, DECEMBER 4, 2013

I HAVE FOUND IT HELPFUL and even entertaining to let my "holy imagination" roam for those precious twelve or so minutes of daily radiation treatment. Yesterday my thoughts drifted to the men (and women) behind the curtain. I first gave thanks to God for the technicians in their cockpit behind that three-foot lead wall, pushing the buttons and running the computer program that governs the radiation delivery apparatus. I appreciated the physicists and dosimetrists who had programmed my treatment protocol, then moved on to give thanks for the machine's manufacturer and all its employees. I thought about the company of researchers and scientists who, over the years, have unpacked the complexities of this disease. While I was at it, I gave thanks for the pharmaceutical companies that have developed drugs to kill it. By the end of this exercise, my mind's eye beheld thousands of people who had been at work for decades in order that I, at that moment, might receive treatment. It was quite a sight!

Every Christian has access to such a group of contributors and should think about them often. The writer of Hebrews underwent this exercise in Hebrews 11, enumerating generation after generation of faithful men and women who had believed God and acted accordingly throughout biblical history. Known in Hebrews 12 as "the great cloud of witnesses," this spiritual cheering section is rooting for every one of us who have trusted Jesus Christ and put our full faith in God's purposes. The present generation of Christians is here because of the courageous witness of someone in generations past. One of Billy Graham's great stories recounts the line of individual evangelists who had led his spiritual forebears to Christ. The last of those was Mordecai Ham, who was gripped by the gospel and commissioned by it to Charlotte, North Carolina, where Graham sank to his knees at a revival meeting.

In some parts of the world, one's list of spiritual forebears includes martyrs whose deaths gave rise to faith among witnesses. There is no other explanation for the expansion of Christianity in China, which within my lifetime was perceived to be a remnant. What we know now is that as a result of the faithful seed planting of missionaries 175 years ago, an underground—albeit persecuted—indigenous church has grown to become a significant presence in that country.

According to Hebrews 12, the role of these spiritual forebears is to cheer us on as we now "run the race set before us." They encourage us to persevere when our lungs are giving out, when our legs are tired, when we are about to give up mentally, when we forget what Christ did to save us. These saints, by their faithful witness, remind us that we are not the first to run this particular race, nor are we the first to suffer or to find it difficult. We are not the first to struggle with giving thanks in our circumstances, nor are we the first to face death. We are only the latest of a long line of ancestors whose battle against God's opponents has taken many forms. They witnessed either the defeat of evil or the hope of same, and their cheers are meant to keep us focused on the finish line, whence we too will urge the next generation to endure its own contest.

I hope in some small way to give courage to someone who is facing his or her own Beast. Think of me as cheering you on. You can do it, with Jesus's help! I'm here to tell you, Jesus Christ has done everything possible to bring you home safely. He suffered and died for you, and by his scourging you were healed! Believe it and keep running (or walking or staggering) toward his finish line. You are not alone on the track. It may feel like you are isolated in your struggle and the saints are but fictional men and women behind the curtain. But Jesus is carrying you to the race's end and will get you to the finish line in one piece, while the rest of us break into boisterous singing to praise him and to greet you!

34

Thinking outside the Pool

THURSDAY, DECEMBER 5, 2013

A S YESTERDAY PROGRESSED I ENJOYED more strength and energy than I have experienced in a few weeks. A sunny, lovely day beckoned me outside. In response to Andy's request, if I was up to it, I could water our orange trees as insurance against an expected overnight freeze. Two weeks ago a slow stroll out to the fig tree was enough to put me down for a nap afterward. This week I have been able to walk all the way around our block, almost three-quarters of a mile, and still be functional afterward. I am coughing very little now, and even the esophageal discomfort (collateral damage of radiation) has quieted. Many people are praying for tolerance of the treatments and for healing. It is also likely—eleven days out from my last chemo treatment—that my body is undergoing its expected recovery from the toxic onslaught.

It surprised me to realize that, after weeks of feeling unwell and deeply tired and reluctantly accepting my new normal, at least for a few months, I had no plan for what to do if I actually felt better. I had no to-do list at the ready, no next steps. I have considered it a necessary and liberating spiritual exercise to learn how to rest, feel useless, wait, and endure. What I encountered from the Lord yesterday was an invitation to be mentally alert, emotionally ready, and spiritually empowered for activity if and when he gives me a fresh wind of healing.

This is a faith issue. The question Jesus is asking is this: If I were to heal you right this minute, what would you do as a result? Have you envisioned what life is going to be like without the weight of cancer on your shoulders? Are you ready to step into the realities and responsibilities that physical health makes possible?

Jesus asks a critical question of the man by the pool at the Sheep's Gate. For thirty-eight years, amid "many invalids—blind, lame, and paralyzed," this poor guys has waited his turn for a healing dip. So Jesus asks, "Do you want to be made well?" (John 5:2–9). You'd think the answer would be obvious, but Jesus had to ask so the man would be mentally prepared for able-bodied life. After thirty-eight years, it was time to think outside the pool.

On a practical level, what does the gift of faith look like? Twenty years ago I worked alongside a gentleman, an elder of our congregation, who was the chairman of the building committee. Our church was planning a building expansion, a process that took over eight years of this man's retirement to accomplish. For years, the town's red tape and the neighbors' protests stalled our ground breaking, causing the price tag to almost double in the meantime.

Mr. Jones was a man of great faith, exhibited by a rich prayer life and divine patience. He was also always ready, at a moment's notice, to take the next step if and when it was allowed by the city. Many decision points were scheduled on the town council's calendar, and you could count on Mr. Jones to have the money, the equipment, and the personnel in place the next day if he got the green light. More often than not, he got a red light. But no one will forget the Tuesday night the town council finally gave approval; Mr. Jones was waving in a huge earthmover on Wednesday morning. That man had faith and he had vision, and I learned a big life lesson from him. Assume that God is going to answer your prayer, and be ready to move into the reality he creates!

35 ✧

Sweet Hour of Prayer and
an Interesting Doctor's Visit

FRIDAY, DECEMBER 6, 2013

MY BODY HAS HAD A chance to recover from the chemical onslaught, and I am amazed at how few side effects I am experiencing. Increased energy has allowed me to participate in a few household pursuits; I even went to the grocery store on my own yesterday. Reminders of sickness are only an occasional cough and fatigue that necessitates a nap. As I feel better and the disciplines of treatment proceed uneventfully, Jesus feels somewhat distant, and the sensation of spiritual acuity has left me—with a notable exception:

My friend and colleague, Tim, offered to take me on a field trip yesterday. He came to pick me up for the thirty-minute drive to a prayer meeting in Livermore. I thought we were going to a church, but our destination was actually the chapel service at Shepherd's Gate, a Christian residential ministry for women at risk. Most of the other attendees were twenty-something women who have found refuge from domestic violence, homelessness, or other crises. They can reside up to eighteen months in this positive, loving environment.

Tim says, "Jesus tends to show up on Thursday mornings as they pray for healing." It was such a sweet time. Their prayers were powerful and earnest, coming from people who are desperately dependent on

Jesus. One of the young residents, Denise, gave me a Scripture the Lord laid on her heart, which I will treasure: "Do not fear, for I am with you, do not be afraid, for I am your God; I will strengthen you, I will help you, I will uphold you with my victorious right hand" (Isa. 41:10).

Another resident, Heidi, offered a personal prayer as she gripped my hands. These women were so deeply grateful for Jesus's transformation in their lives, and I was moved by their burning desire to pass God's blessing on to me—they were blessed to be a blessing (Gen. 12:1–3).

My health condition didn't change; I felt no immediate, miraculous healing. But God was healing in that room, and I left with a song in my heart and gratitude for the answers to prayer I have already experienced: cessation of the cough, healing of my esophageal discomfort a week ago, the calming of my gut, and the relational riches that surround me.

This morning after my radiation treatment, I had my weekly sit-down with Dr. Rahman, the radiation oncologist. She was delighted to see how well I was doing and said my blood work seems on track for this stage of treatment. She is quite sure my overall health, strength, and "clean living" have set me up to respond well to treatment. I was thinking, *This treatment regimen is going to be a piece of cake.*

But she went on. "You feel really good now, but round two of chemo is going to hit you pretty hard. I want you to be prepared."

As I filed that uncomfortable forecast away, we discussed the next steps of treatment. Dr. Rahman said, "After round two is complete, right before Christmas, we're going to assess tumor shrinkage. If you are making progress, then surgery would be the next step, if you choose it. Just in case you opt out of surgery, or if there is more to be done to reduce the tumor, we will have a new radiation treatment plan designed and ready to implement. That way there won't be any gaps in your treatment schedule to slow down the momentum."

In the course of our conversation, a fact forgotten along the way gave me a momentary shock: the PET scan weeks ago showed cancer in *three* lymph nodes, not just the one that was biopsied. To Dr. Rahman this was old news, and all treatment plans had taken this into account from the beginning.

Would knowing the cancer had penetrated three lymph nodes have changed my outlook on my cancer? I have gone this long without worrying about it. Nothing good would come of more anxiety now. The radiation is directed at all three lymph nodes and has been from the beginning. The situation has not changed, allowing me to proceed on the established treatment path without further worry.

What confidence I have comes from a bedrock belief: from day to day my circumstances might change, or *not*, but God remains the same (Heb. 13:8). God renews his tender mercies every morning (Lam. 3:23); his character is steadfast and immovable—always good, always loving, always redeeming, always attentive (Ps. 145); and nothing can wrest me from his arms (Rom. 8:37–39). God was taking care of me before I learned of my cancer, and he is taking care of me still. Nothing about my situation is news to him, and he is taking the necessary steps to address my condition, whether I am aware or not.

The great privilege we have is to experience God's gracious arms holding us steadfast. The slaying of the Beast will come at the right time, with the sweep of God's mighty hand. In the meantime that same God is with us, with promises of strength and help through the days when "no change" is the reality. To our unchanging God be the glory!

36 ✍

Collateral Damage

LUNG CANCER LIKE MINE REQUIRES aggressive treatment. In my case it involves both chemotherapy and radiation, designed to shrink the tumor to a size that can be excised safely and to kill any rogue cells that might be migrating through my body. The medicines in my chemo infusions have a proven track record, and the presurgery treatment protocol is noncontroversial. But collateral damage makes the regimen tough on the body.

In a military context, *collateral damage* is a sterile term for the death or injury of innocent bystanders. Medically, it refers to the damage radiation can cause to healthy tissues that are not the primary target—skin, normal lung tissue, and esophagus, through which radiation beams travel to reach the tumor. Chemo puts a strain on the kidneys, nerves, and blood formation, eventually suppressing my immunity.

Those consent forms I signed a few weeks ago acknowledged the possible side effects of treatment. I calculated the risks and deemed them worth taking. Killing the Beast—and thereby saving my life—was the primary objective. I hope the collateral damage will prove to be insignificant compared to the benefits of living without cancer.

In the Christian life, we can expect collateral damage when we resist temptation and push back on sin. The writer of Hebrews honestly addresses this dynamic and presents us with a challenge: "Consider [Jesus] who endured such hostility against himself from sinners, so that you may not grow weary or lose heart. In your struggle against sin you have not yet resisted to the point of shedding your blood" (Heb. 12:3–4).

Forsaking sin might make us bleed! For example, removing ourselves from tempting situations might require leaving friends closely associated with bad habits. What could be more painful than that? Only the alienation from God brought on by the sinful practice. And yet, how often are we deceived into thinking it is more important or loving to keep a friend or a job or a habit than to finally wriggle free of the immoral trap that has been set for us? More likely, how often are we lulled into thinking that continuing in sin really isn't hurting us and it isn't worth the pain of extricating ourselves from it?

And yet, if Jesus had thought that way, he would have given up the idea of carrying the cross, suffering the pain and shame of execution. He could have said, in the flesh, "This dying is just too much trouble; and for what? To redeem hopeless, sinful people who have forsaken their heavenly Father?"

But no, Jesus willingly took on the one and only remedy for our hopelessness and sin, his own death on our behalf. Again, in Hebrews 12:2: "[Look] to Jesus, the pioneer and perfecter of our faith, who for the sake of the joy that was set before him endured the cross, disregarding its shame."

To illustrate, pastors pay a high price to remain faithful in moments when parishioners come to them toe-to-toe with some sort of ultimatum. Early in my tenure as a senior pastor, a long-standing church member—known to be a manipulator and power grabber—came to my office to offer a large sum of money to the church. In order to get an end-of-year tax deduction, he was legally required to give the gift without designation, but he wanted a verbal agreement that the funds would be spent on his pet project, which even I recognized would divert the focus of our ministry. I explained that I could not make such a commitment without the participation of our board of elders—a cop-out answer, I know—to buy me some time to sort out why I felt so uncomfortable with the overture. I ended up declining his gift out of concern it would forge an unholy alliance with an individual whose aims were not consistent with the church's mission. With a great harrumph he "took his money elsewhere" and made my life miserable for the next two years until he transferred membership to another church. The entire episode came at a high cost to me emotionally and to the church financially. But whatever we lost to collateral damage was gained in future years as the elders stood strong in wisdom and faithfulness.

Jesus spilled his own blood, and by that action poured out his forgiveness and empowered us to forsake the sinful actions that entangle us in unholy living. Nobody said this forsaking business would be pretty; in fact, we are promised it will be painful. And yet, "to those who are trained by [that discipline], later it yields the peaceful fruit of righteousness" (Heb. 12:11). The collateral damage to our pride and our wayward relationships and habits is a necessary part of our repentance. If we remain strong in the Lord and healthy in our faith, we can withstand the side effects of deep and true repentance, as painful as they are.

Following Jesus this day could be difficult; we must keep our eyes on him and not be diverted from the path of righteousness. Saying "yes" to Jesus today will require saying "no" to temptation or sin that has already entangled us. May God give us the wisdom to choose rightly and courageously, despite the short-term pain. The long-term gain is joyful fellowship with our heavenly Father and demonstrating the power of his kingdom to the world around us!

37 ✍

Serendipity

Tuesday, December 10, 2013, 5 a.m.

CANCER TREATMENT INEVITABLY BRINGS ON collateral damage, negative consequences of an action meant to do good. But it is also accompanied by serendipity: the finding of valuable or agreeable things not sought for. The Post-it Note is a famous case of serendipity. The 3M Company, formulating a new adhesive and encountering one failure after another, discovered a compound that became a temporary glue.

Some surprising side benefits have accompanied my chemotherapy: the steroid that amps up the antinausea medicine has relieved the pain of my March shoulder injury, so I now have full range of motion. My limited stamina has called forth the companionship of a parade of friends who sit with me each afternoon for quality, faith-building conversation. The cough that originally announced the presence of the Beast is almost gone. For some reason my metabolism is accelerated, and I can eat anything I want, anytime, without gaining weight. And certainly I have precious hours of quiet time each day in which to listen to God, write, and sew.

Serendipity is embedded in the biblical story of Joseph and his brothers in Genesis. As a young whippersnapper, Joseph had a pride problem, and his eleven brothers were sick of it. Joseph was a favored son and had received a special gift of a multicolored coat. He flaunted his status before his brothers, who decided one day to give him his comeuppance. They stripped him, threw him into a cistern to die, smeared animal blood on the coat, and took it to their father as evidence that Joseph was dead. An unthinkable thing to do to a brother and a father!

Meanwhile, an Ishmaelite caravan passed by. Jacob's opportunistic sons saw that they could profit by a more creative approach. They hauled their brother out of the pit and sold him to the traders for twenty pieces of silver. Joseph was carted off to Egypt and sold into slavery. Over time he matured and his gifts emerged. A remarkable transformation put him in a position of incredible power in that country. Near the end of the story, his brothers, suffering through a famine in Israel, came to Egypt for foreign aid. They did not recognize Joseph, who staged a dramatic reveal and provided the whole Jacob clan safe haven.

In the final great scene of this saga, after Jacob had died and the brothers feared Joseph's revenge, Joseph declared to them: "Look, you perpetrated a great evil upon me and meant to harm me. But God meant it for good, so that his people could be preserved" (Gen. 50:20, *my paraphrase*). That is serendipity of the highest order: "You intended evil, but God meant it for good."

One way of looking at my illness (and whatever trial *you* may be going through) is to recognize that Satan intends destruction, but God is working his redemptive kingdom purposes. This powerful reality helps me to live in hope that God will indeed bring good out of a bad situation, to see ministry potential in suffering, and to give God glory and praise. The balm this is to my spirit cannot be measured.

38

Loss of Hair

TUESDAY, DECEMBER 10, 2013, 4 P.M.

MY HAIR STARTED TO FALL out yesterday, right on schedule, three weeks exactly after my first chemo treatment. I secretly hoped I would be an exception to the norm. However, now that hair loss is happening, I am more amused than upset. What caught my attention first was the feeling I had put on a shirt worn during a haircut. Then, after my walk, my fleece hat held a soft nest of loose hairs. This morning in the shower, tresses cascaded down my face. Laughing, I called out to my husband, "I'm shedding like a dog!"

The last straw was finding hair strands in my casserole leftovers at lunch. Oh, bother.

Tonight I will consult with Andy about next measures: shave it off to avoid the mess? Wrap it up in a scarf? Or just keep vacuuming?

I haven't decided about a wig yet. Most women I have talked to say their wigs were scratchy and uncomfortable on a sensitive scalp. Perhaps it would be beneficial to check out the local nonprofit that provides free wigs to women with cancer. If I find something I like, I have a back-up plan. Otherwise, colorful headscarves will express my personality just fine.

39 ✑

Making Things Happen vs.
Letting Things Happen

WEDNESDAY, DECEMBER 11, 2013, 5:15 A.M.

I HAVE NOW EXPERIENCED LOSS of control over something as simple as grooming.

The hair fall this week reminded me of the difference between *making* things happen and *letting* things happen. I worked with a pastor once who believed leaders must *make* things happen. This philosophy of ministry manifested itself in meticulous planning, control over every step of a process, forceful persuasion to his point of view, and tireless labor. Aside from resulting in a driven personality, this approach did not leave room for God to work. To let things happen was tantamount to giving up, admitting defeat, and abdicating responsibility. He believed one must never relinquish control over a situation.

Leadership requires the kind of focus I have just described in certain times and situations, but we must keep a few eternal truths in mind as we barrel forward. The illusion that we can control everything and everyone as we exercise leadership is folly relationally, physically, and spiritually.

Relational folly. By its very nature, the drive to control involves controlling people, not just processes. There is a fine line between godly shepherding, which does involve a rod and staff every once in a while, and coercion, which forces a leader's will upon another. In the church, not only do we want to get things done, but we also want to participate in the people-shaping process of discipleship. The goal is not to bend people to *my* will but to encourage an atmosphere in which we all, together, submit to *God's* will. The relationship between Christian leader and follower requires even the leader to view herself as a follower of Jesus, pointing others to the Good Shepherd. This approach allows pastor and layperson to relate authentically and humbly, engaging in the mutual submission that is to characterize our life together (Eph. 5:20).

Further, if my focus is on making things happen, relationships very easily turn into utilitarian arrangements. As long as other people are useful to the task, a "relationship" exists. But if they flake or chafe or show creativity in a direction that doesn't fit my agenda, the relationship wanes.

Physical folly. I have seen control freaks all too often crash and burn from the burden of holding everything together. It is not good for the body. Controlling everything going on around you is exhausting. As a young pastor going through a burnout phase myself, I remember planning into my schedule a monthly all-nighter to meet a newsletter deadline. The choice I made, in retrospect, was not only a self-inflicted violation of boundaries, but also an unsustainable work pattern. Granted, certain seasons in the church year require extra effort, but if one violates one's sabbath on a regular basis under the banner of making things happen, a line has been crossed.

Spiritual folly. But really, what does it say about our relationship with God that *we* must make everything happen? Are we responding to God's sovereign authority in the midst of life's challenges, or are we competing for power? If making things happen means telling God what is to unfold and how, we have reversed the roles and taken unto ourselves what is rightfully God's. Psalm 46:10 (NASB) says, "Cease striving, and know that I am God!" And from Proverbs: "The human mind plans the way, but the Lord directs the steps" (16:9). Our planning efforts must never trump the Lord's direction.

Years ago I arrived at a new call and discovered that the church-sponsored nursery school was not overtly Christian in its orientation. Seeing this as a missed opportunity, I set a goal to change it. But very clearly God said to me, "Mary, I want you to wait. I am going to take care of this situation myself, and I want you to stand back and watch what I do." So that task fell to the bottom of my Things To Do list. Within a year or two the director resigned, and we were able to select a wonderful new leader to set a new direction. The transition was (almost) painless, organic, and smooth and bore much fruit in the years to come. All I had to do was let it happen in God's good timing.

As for the head-shaving, to continue the illustration (but not to prescribe what you should do in a similar situation): I could have made things happen by shaving my head two weeks ago, before hair fall was certain. Now that the process is actually underway, I am invited to accept it and deal with it appropriately. Shaving my head now saves the inevitable mess of a clogged shower drain and the discomfort of hair in my shirt. But whatever I do, I believe that God, who can lovingly account for every hair on my head, is directing my steps. It is my desire not to seize control but to follow those directions well and to lead others to the One who really does make things happen.

40 ✍

I Should Have My Head Examined

WEDNESDAY, DECEMBER 11, 2013, 10 P.M.

WHEN ANDY GOT HOME FROM work, I asked him to shave my head. Two friends came over for moral support, which Andy needed more than I did. "Dear, this is the hardest thing I have ever done for you." We tried to have some fun with it by shaving strips off in stages and taking pictures: the monk, the Mohawk, the Elmer Fudd. And then, at last, I could examine the shape of my head—not bad!

I have an appointment to check out wigs on Friday morning, and hats are on the way from family members who think it's the perfect time for me to support their sports teams.

A long time ago, a friend with a brain tumor told me, "If you can't fix it, feature it." Hair loss is a done deal; I can't fix that. But I can express myself with colorful scarves and cute hats in the jewel-tone colors I love. My friend, Viola, has sent me my first infinity scarf for a Hollywood starlet look. I feel armed and dangerous!

41 ✐

I Have a Friend

A TINGLY HEAD, HAIRY SHIRT collars, and patches of bare scalp made shaving off my locks inevitable and necessary. When I told my friends my plan, Sandi piped up. "I will shave my head too. What time should I come over?"

Astounded, and concerned for her welfare in winter, I tried to talk her out of it. But she was resolute. So at 8:00 p.m. last night, Sandi and her husband Jim came knocking cheerfully at our door, and out came the hair clippers. By 9:30 we were both as bald as newborn babies.

Friendship takes many forms, and this elegant act of solidarity by a sister is a fine example. The outpouring of love and practical help by my friends in the last few weeks has been heartening and at times moving. Yesterday Sarah sat with me; our afternoon's conversation yielded spiritual encouragement and the discovery of many common interests, experiences, and elements of family background.

At this time of Advent, I am reminded of a kinship that encouraged two women surprised by unfolding circumstances in their lives. The maiden Mary had been visited by an angel telling her she would conceive by the Holy Spirit a child who would be Son of God. And oh, by the way, your cousin, Elizabeth, who was barren, is also with child! So Mary, for reasons not given in Luke 1, where this account appears, dashes off to the hill country to visit her relative. When the two women meet, blessings are exchanged, and even the next generation they bear rises in joyful greeting. They stay together in mutual support and solidarity for three months, after which Mary returns to her hometown to await the birth of our Savior (Luke 1:24–56).

The gift of friendship, expressed as *koinonia* within the Christian community, is a lifeline for people who otherwise would feel alone with their maladies, surprises, temptations, and personal triumphs. Pastors need friends too, but they are often isolated by their position and the inherent power dynamic that necessitates boundaries with parishioners. Some pastors shun close friendships altogether, either because they are too busy to pursue relationships with people outside their congregation or because they are afraid to be known. To them I say, find out who your true friends are, cherish them, and let them hold you accountable to an authentic Christian life even while "off duty."

For all of us, friendship is not a luxury but a necessity. And I am not talking about electronic social networks. My daughters needed to see me face to face at Thanksgiving, despite our regular texting and phone conversations over the previous three weeks. They needed to see in my eyes that I was not faking joviality on the phone or otherwise obscuring my true condition.

A personal visit is worth a thousand texts. If you hesitate to make that effort out of concerns about what to say, what you might see, or how they might react, then ask for that wonderful Jesus-compassion that sees through bald heads to buffeted hearts. Shortly after I entered the ministry, a church member asked if I would visit a cancer patient with my guitar and sing her a couple songs. At the time, young and inexperienced as I was, I could not see myself doing that. I was afraid. I didn't even know what I was afraid of, but I didn't go. I knew this refusal represented a failure, or an immaturity, so I asked God to work in me.

Since then I have visited countless parishioners and have even been present at the time of death. I have discovered the joyful, holy moments that come with standing alongside people at their weakest. All that experience visiting others has certainly prepared me for my own limp-along journey now. And my friends are showing me the grace and generosity that are strengthening my spirit and helping me to rest in Jesus.

It is Jesus, ultimately, who says to us, "You've got a friend . . . all you have to do is call my name!" Often that friend shows up wearing your sunny face, bearing your yummy dinner, or bringing up interesting topics in the course of your conversation. For this I am deeply grateful.

42 ✑

The Backstory for a Big Decision

YESTERDAY WAS A BUSY AND informative day: radiation at 8:40, then weekly checkups with both medical oncology and radiation oncology, and finally a trip to The Wig Source, a local nonprofit that supplies wigs to cancer patients who have lost their hair.

My radiation oncologist, Dr. Sophia Rahman, spent forty minutes with me discussing background information I will need for a big decision coming up. At the end of this week, I will have received the 45-Gray dose of radiation appropriate for preoperative shrinkage of a tumor. By Monday, December 23, I will have completed the second chemo cycle. The question will be, has the tumor decreased in size and retreated from aorta, windpipe, and esophagus enough that it can be taken out safely? The CT scan of the region will be done on December 19, and all will be discussed and decided with the surgeon on December 24. (Merry Christmas!)

The size and position of the tumor could prevent the surgeon from extricating it from its very delicate position in my upper left lobe. Then, instead of surgery, chemotherapy would continue and a "definitive dose" of radiation (up to 60-Gray) would be administered in the next two weeks. That higher dose of radiation disqualifies me from surgery because it compromises the tissue's ability to heal. Fortunately, this choice is as effective as surgery; the old, dead tumor just gradually dissolves, and its dead cells are sloughed off through normal systems in the body. They call that option "curative."

Surgery would provide me with a statistically insignificant advantage over the radiation option: the Beast would be gone for good, and I would be able to avoid further radiation side effects. However, I would also lose the entire upper left lobe of my lung, which deserves some consideration since singing is an important part of my life.

No decision can be made without the surgeon's evaluation of the CT scan, but we must resolve the question in a timely manner to prevent any interruption to my treatment. The oncologist and the surgeon wanted me to have the broader context that informs the decision so I won't have to process everything in one day. I love the fact that the doctors decided together that I should get this information now and chew on it for a week.

Daughter Judy has just arrived for a long holiday stay so we can discuss my options face to face.

43 ✿

Freedom in Confinement

THE NEWS THIS WEEK HAS been dominated by the death of Nelson Mandela and the celebrations of his life. His greatness is measured by the impact of his personal transformation on a nation sullied by apartheid. His vocal and powerful political advocacy prior to his incarceration was supposedly silenced by imprisonment; but, as we all know, his was a witness of presence in his absence. His body was in the dungeon, so to speak, but his will and his spirit escaped into the conscience of a country and the world.

The most remarkable feature of his life was what he did after he was released. He forgave his captors and reached across the great racial divide to unite a nation and form a new government. Trading anger for reconciliation is the great work of personal transformation for which he will be known, and it was those decades in prison that accomplished it.

Lifelong Methodist missionary to India E. Stanley Jones once observed, "[If] you are not able to get out of the dungeon, then the only thing to do is to get the dungeon out of you—to find grace in that very dungeon."[5]

When harbored resentment or anger binds us more tightly than prison walls, we confine ourselves in a dungeon of our own making. In my case, I could view my illness and fatigue as a prison preventing me from doing what I love to do. For you, the prison might be a life in hyperdrive, leaving no time for reflection or recreation. For someone else, the dungeon might be a dark hole of addiction. We all have life circumstances or conditions that might, if we let them, imprison us. The challenge is to examine those limitations in a different light.

We are helped by reflecting on individuals in the Bible who themselves were imprisoned. The Old Testament portrays Joseph in an Egyptian prison (Gen. 37 and following). In Acts Paul and Silas were thrown into jail because their preaching in Philippi ruffled enough feathers to induce the magistrates to arrest them for disturbing the peace. Paul and Silas responded in an unexpected way: "About midnight Paul and Silas were praying and singing hymns to God, and the prisoners were listening to them" (Acts 16:22–25).

Even though the two evangelists were beaten and chained, worship transported them into the presence of God. Their bodies were locked in the stocks, but their unconfined spirits soared.

Paul and Silas inspire me to think differently about physical freedom and confinement, about the possibilities for meaningful activity even when limited to my chemo chair for more than five hours today. It helps, I acknowledge, that I have chosen this temporary discipline of limited mobility in order to experience full freedom later. But I also recognize how easily one's essential identity can morph from "healthy and free" to "ill and limited."

The challenge is to keep God's vision for my life before me. At the very least, my heavenly citizenship allows me to enjoy full access to God in prayer, full reign in God's kingdom to minister in my new context, full freedom to dream and imagine and write as God inspires me. Jesus himself is the finest illustration of one who could not be confined, even to the grave. To choose life despite limitations is to dwell in resurrection hope, following in the footsteps of our Savior and his saints. It is more than making lemonade out of life's lemons; it is abiding in Jesus Christ and sharing his vision of "the joy set before him" (Heb. 12:2), even as he suffered. I choose to live in this kind of joyful emancipation today.

44 ✑

A Long Obedience in a (Tedious) Direction

TUESDAY, DECEMBER 17, 2013

THE EARLY NOVELTY OF ENTERING into treatment for lung cancer has worn off, though I remain steadfastly focused on healing. This week I entered round two of chemotherapy, while continuing with daily radiation. No new drama or new happenings or side effects of note.

Life's routine can put us in a pattern of activity and behavior that is boring. Perhaps I am bringing this up at the wrong time of year. Holiday event schedules might be too crazy to even think about spiritual things right now. But let's say life is marching along predictable paths, requiring a daily slog through the bog of known responsibilities, offering no immediate reward, affirmation, or excitement. A period like this requires what Eugene Peterson called "a long obedience in the same direction."

I have been reflecting on the long trek of the Israelites after the excitement of their escape across the Red Sea (Ex. 14) and after the manna routine had settled in (Ex. 16). What I see is a wilderness fraught with temptations all the more alluring, given the tedious nature of their task. How many of these lurk at the edges of our long obedience?

The Temptation to Go Back to the "Before" Life (Ex. 15:22–16:3). Once the realities of life in the wilderness sank in, the Israelites actually entertained the lie that they had it better under slavery in Egypt, forgetting that for centuries they had been oppressed and exploited.

On my personal timeline, I now refer to BC (Before Cancer) and AD (After Diagnosis); the BC days were sweet, energetic, celebratory, and productive. The devil would like me to believe that the current AD days *cannot* be sweet, powerful, joyful, and even productive. But I enjoy all those gifts now because God himself is present and generous with his love expressed through his people.

The Temptation to Grumble (Num. 14). As heavy burdens of wilderness life settled upon them, the Israelites started turning on Moses and complaining night and day about his leadership, about the conditions, about their hunger and thirst. They were not happy campers, literally. If I were to grumble about details of daily life (and there are certainly opportunities to do so), I would simply be squandering the opportunities to return thanks and meditate on God's goodness and strength, while spurning the considerable resources gathered to achieve my healing.

The Temptation to Make Things Happen (Ex. 32). When Moses took off to climb Mount Sinai, his departure was not without some explanation and fanfare. He was going into the smoke, fire, and thunder of the peak to meet God. The people were told to keep a safe distance and to wait, presumably for some revelation when Moses returned. But gee, he's been gone for forty days, and we think he has ditched us, and here we are out in the middle of nowhere with no leader, no God, and no entertainment. Hearing their complaints, Aaron has a brilliant idea.[6] He tells the people to throw all their gold into the fire to melt it, and then he fashions a "golden calf," an idol that becomes the honored guest at one heck of a party. *(I want to know where they got the mold.)* The real temptation when life gets predictable and boring is to elevate an idol around which something interesting might happen. My computer, or the food I can still taste, or *Downton Abbey* reruns can all take on idol status. Whatever it is, if it competes for God's exalted position in my life, it must be kept in its place through discipline and wisdom and a long obedience empowered by the ever-present Holy Spirit.

So on this new day, despite its tedium, I would like to recognize the temptations before I fall into their traps. I want to do what is necessary—avert a gaze, turn off a machine, address the needs of others—to walk toward God, who has held me upright on this cancer road and keeps me going in the right direction. Asking myself these questions periodically helps: 1) How is God working his purposes in the midst of my suffering?; 2) Am I on board with what God is trying to do in me and through me?; and 3) In what way can I show my gratitude today?

45 ✍

Living Water Keeps Flowing

At least once a week a surprise package arrives in the mail or lands on my front porch. These random acts of kindness come from friends far and near who have sent not a Christmas present but an "open me now" gift of encouragement. Honestly, I am put to shame for lack of creativity in all these years of walking alongside buddies who have had cancer or some other life-altering medical condition.

Just a sampling: Emily sent a pair of cashmere socks I wear all the time now. Viola sent two headscarves, one so clever I had to call her for instructions on how to wear it. Church elders sent a gorgeous calligraphy rendering of Aaron's blessing: "The Lord bless you and keep you; the Lord make his face to shine upon you, and be gracious to you; the Lord lift up his countenance upon you, and give you peace" (Num. 6:24–26). My anonymous "coffee angel" delivers a half pound of my favorite decaf every Tuesday; Randy sends a funny or heartwarming video each Friday. A church member brought a huge poinsettia for the front porch. The list goes on, but the effect is the same: The great blessing that has been flowing in my direction since the end of October reminds and convinces me that I am not alone, that I am loved, and that I have many people praying for me.

It would be easy to develop a sense of entitlement and to hoard the proceeds of illness. In particular, I feel little desire or obligation to share the premium chocolate bar Louise sent me, because it's mine and chocolate is medicine, right? I could follow in Israel's footsteps and believe only in my chosen-ness and not in any commission to be a light in the world or a supporter of the poor (flaws revealed by the biblical prophets).

Andy came home from work last night with a lousy head cold. My beloved, who has been tender and merciful, generous and self-giving, patient and tolerant of my limitations, now is weak and contagious and needing help. It is my turn to return the blessing. And how grateful I am that last evening I had a surge of energy to complete tasks that ordinarily would belong to him in our new household order: doing a load of laundry, emptying the dishwasher, getting the house ready for a thorough cleaning today. Given my compromised immune system, it also meant sleeping in my recliner instead of in bed next to him, but this too was God's unglamorous opportunity for me to be a blessing.

When Jesus called himself the living water, he was invoking a strong mental image of a Jewish custom. The *mikvah* bath prepares every Jewish male for worship, and the water source must be "living"; that is, it must flow from a clean source, through the bath facility, and outside, to carry away uncleanness. Jesus, the living water, washes us with God's unlimited supply of forgiveness and grace. And in Abrahamic "blessed to be a blessing" fashion, the blessing we receive is intended to wash through us into the lives of others. If the blessing stops with us, we become a cistern of stinky selfishness with a mistaken notion of entitlement.

We must resist the temptation to hoard our blessings. We have been blessed to be a blessing, so we keep it moving, in living water fashion, so others can know the love of God through us today.

46 🖋

Living in Suspense

THURSDAY, DECEMBER 19, 2013

ONE OF THE PLEASURES OF a quiet life and hours in the chemo chair each day is recreational reading. Right now it's a legal thriller called *Havana Requiem* by Paul Goldstein. This tightly written novel by the Stanford author unfolds in Grisham style to reveal the rich tapestry of pre- and post-revolution Cuba. The suspenseful tale leads to musical discoveries of cultural significance and, in typical murder mystery style, "a body in the library."

You can imagine my consternation when I turn page 216 to find I am back on page 154. Flipping through, I realize an entire leaf of the book is defective, repeating previous pages and missing every even-numbered page of the book's conclusion! Now I am *really* in suspense and scrambling for a quick fix.

But hold on a moment; this mildly frustrating experience invites me to examine the suspenseful life I am leading this season. Along with What will Santa bring me this year? I am dealing with much bigger questions: How successful will my cancer treatment be? Which of two mutually exclusive approaches to slaying the Beast should I choose next week? When will I be able to go back to work?

The people of God have lived in suspense almost from the very beginning of time. In the Garden of Eden, this suspense took the form of delightful anticipation of discovery amid a wonderful creation. After the fall, many other features of life became unknown—dark and threatening to humanity's well-being. Abraham was held in suspense when God said, "Come with me to a land I will show you," and Abe followed without knowing where he was going. We certainly see excitement and suspense in the Israelites' outrunning their Egyptian pursuers across the Red Sea and in the forty years of wandering in the desert, wondering what the land of milk and honey looked like. As the New Testament opens, we see Simeon and Anna longing for the Savior, and we watch their faces as they greet Mary and her baby Jesus: "Ah, now your servant can depart in peace." The people of God are in suspense—we could also call it faith—because we live hoping to see the mighty hand of God at work. Ultimately, we await the second coming of the Lord Jesus Christ and the resolution of all that is unfinished and yet to be redeemed.

What fuels our hope is the benevolent and faithful foundation God has already laid. We need to turn *back* the pages and recall what God has done. Throughout the Old Testament, the Israelites are commanded to tell their story over and over again: of the Exodus, of their forebears in faith, of the ordered life described in the Law of God. As they return from Babylonian exile, Ezra and Nehemiah lead the people in reading the Law for days and teaching one another what it means for their life together in the future. And we, in the long line of apostles and teachers and disciples of Christ, read and reread the Scriptures, Jesus's Word of life, to anchor our future in a faithful history with God.

As I embark upon the next few days of investigation and decision-making, God is reminding me to hold fast to the parts of my story already known and experienced. My written cancer chronicle over the last few weeks is helping me remember God's presence in my treatment, the shower of blessings from friends, and the love and support of my family. Turning back the pages, I know that God has never left me, that he is carrying me, and that his people have my back, even when I am too tired to pray. I know God has power; he has held back serious side effects of treatment and kept me comfortable through chemo and radiation. All along he has been guiding me, steering me out of trouble, and otherwise keeping me on his path toward healing. These are the truths I embrace, even as I face the suspense of "What is going to happen next."

I may never know how *Havana Requiem* turns out, but I do know that my life is in God's hands and that there is nothing to fear as I live out my story. The suspense itself is exciting and wonderful, because the author of my story has written my name in the Book of Life.

47 ✄

God's Strength When I Am Weak

Friday, December 20, 2013

M Y ENERGY LEVEL IS LOW on days four and five of chemo round two. Have you ever felt tired of being tired? That's where I am today, after a fitful night's sleep.

But a good and logical explanation consoles me. The medicine is a poison slaying the Beast. All my healthy cells are working hard. Radiation is assaulting the intruder, causing some collateral damage in the fray. One of my friends commented, "I'm praying you just get through this, Mary"; this is one of those days simply to endure. The predicted esophageal discomfort from radiation has set in, so I am back on antacids for a week. Soon I will know if I am to continue radiation treatments (with more collateral damage to the esophagus) or prepare for surgery.

Encouragement comes in many forms. Two of my "Peet's ladies" from the local coffee shop stopped by yesterday afternoon for an hour of chatter. I miss our Wednesday coffee klatches so much, but they are keeping the candle lit for me, and I will have the strength to join them in regular fellowship soon. My hammock moment of early November washes over me once again. "Mary, feel this. Feel my presence wrapped around you. I have you in my arms just as surely as this hammock bears your full weight. I am going to carry you through the experience unfolding in your life. Trust me."

The same Shepherd of my soul that made that promise is holding me still today, and I am grateful. I will get through this day only because I will have been carried, not because I have walked in my own strength.

Jesus knew some days would be hard when he gave the invitation: "Come to me, all you that are weary and are carrying heavy burdens, and I will give you rest. Take my yoke upon you, and learn from me; for I am gentle and humble in heart, and you will find rest for your souls. For my yoke is easy, and my burden is light" (Matt. 11:28–30).

This rest fulfills the prophecy of Isaiah, set to music in Handel's *Messiah*: "He will feed his flock like a shepherd; he will gather the lambs in his arms, and carry them in his bosom" (Isa. 40:11).

So let us be carried today by the One who is strong enough to bear our full weight. We shall get through this!

48 &

A Day to Endure

MY ENERGY LEVEL IS TANKING, although nothing about yesterday's radiation and chemo was new. The infusion went well, and this time I was sleepy from the beginning. Might have had something to do with not eating, in preparation for the CT chest scan, scheduled for noon. That procedure went quickly, though, and daughter Judy's grilled cheese sandwich and pot of beef soup went a long way to encourage me afterward.

I had trouble sleeping last night, and for some reason my thoughts went to a dark place. I imagined surrendering and dying, losing the battle, drained of all energy, blind and deaf to the people I love. My chest tightened in anticipation of losing breath, and for a moment all hope for living was lost. I'm still in the dark about my future, and it's probably time to wrestle with death and dying. It really could happen in the next year; I am not in denial about the possibilities this disease holds. But how inconveniently timed are my mental wanderings in the graveyard! Family is gathering for Christmas. The season of noel is upon us. I wish my psyche were on schedule with the church year; isn't death a topic for Lent? Finally, believing my mortality can be taken up another day and having the power to choose what I want to think about, I put these thoughts aside and managed to get back to sleep.

Today may be my last day of radiation. If so, I will miss the chipper tech staff I have met every morning for the last five weeks. If not, this routine continues for another two weeks. On Tuesday we'll know which way we're going. As for chemo, I have the one infusion today, then one more Monday of Cisplatin, and then round two is done. We can do this—with the Lord's strength!

CHRISTMASTIDE

49 ✑

CT Scan Results: Progress to Report!

YESTERDAY WAS MY LAST DAY of radiation. We've reached maximum preoperative dose. Monday is my last chemo treatment of round two. The time has come for a midcourse evaluation of progress by a new CT scan of my chest.

The good news is that the lung tumor has shrunk by over 60 percent! That's almost a two-thirds reduction in two months. And just as side effects of radiation linger for a while after treatment pauses, so does the primary effect—tumor shrinkage. We are on the right trajectory.

What relief! The treatment is working. Now the surgeon must determine whether the tumor has pulled away from the central structures enough to make surgery possible. I will see Dr. Straznicka in three days.

Nothing else shows up on the CT scan. Lymph nodes are of normal size; no other lung nodules in evidence. It seems the cancer has been stopped dead in its tracks, and I am delighted.

50 ✑

Christ Enters My World:
Christmas according to Matthew

PREACHERS HAVE A DUAL CHALLENGE each week: to study a scriptural text for preaching and to interpret where their people are in a position to hear it. Because of my current detachment from my church family for the sake of prudence (avoidance of the colds and flu going around), Christmas seems to be the last thing on my mind these days. I have not seen the decorations in the sanctuary, attended a party, or even completed my Christmas shopping. My mental space is occupied with the decision to be made on the morning of Christmas Eve: Plan A (surgery) or Plan B (no surgery and more radiation).

I woke up early this morning realizing that embracing the holy liturgical season of Christmastide is going to require some spiritual discipline on my part. Somehow I must find a way to integrate my current situation into the narrative of Christmas and bring the Word to *my* life. It is really what we are all called to do as Christians: to answer the question, How does the fact of Christ's birth enter *my* world, even as he entered *the* world? I have decided, in the days between now and Christmas, to look at the birth narrative in each of the four gospels and see what they have to say about life as we are living it.

Only Matthew's account records details surrounding Jesus's birth as seen from Joseph's perspective. The very human concerns about Mary's status as an unwed mother preoccupy Joseph for a while. He, being "a righteous man and unwilling to expose her to public disgrace," planned to divorce her quietly according to Jewish custom (1:19). But before he could carry that out, the angel appeared to him to explain what was going on and what he was to do in order to cooperate with God's strategy. Gabriel's message required Joseph to enter fully into Mary's situation, take her as his wife, and accompany his new family on an unknown journey. After the birth he fulfilled the terms of his assignment, doing as the Lord commanded, and named the baby Jesus, "for he will save his people from their sins" (1:21).

I love the fact that in this rendition of the Christmas story God accounted for the feelings and calling of Joseph and rallied his support for the great redemption project underway. God went to special lengths to secure Joseph's buy-in. Jesus was entering not only Mary's world but also Joseph's; God provided a family of faith to surround the helpless babe and keep him safe. The mission required both adults to listen to God and obey his leading. It required them to take risks together, in this case to flee to Egypt to avoid Herod's murderous intentions. It required them to own the vision God had cast for their son as ruler and shepherd of God's people—a much bigger enterprise than most parents aspire to upon the birth of a firstborn. It required them to hold onto hope of a very big future happening, despite the immediate threat of doom.

This is how Jesus is entering my world and the world of my family these days. God is at work not only in my life but also in my husband's and adult children's lives, enabling us to face our current challenge together. I trust that this experience will enable each of us to draw closer to God and empower us to find joy in the Lord's redemption. We're all going at our own pace, using our own vocabularies, handling difficulties with our unique gifts and perspectives. For this I am so deeply grateful. As I have received my new ministry assignment—to walk this journey with joy and integrity—the "Josephs" in my life have also heard from the Lord a call to be part of the journey. They have rallied already, and it is a joy to experience.

Within a day or two, we will all be together for the week of Christmas.

On Tuesday morning we will huddle together in an examining room to hear what my surgeon has to say about my next steps. God is able to knit our hearts together in common purpose and courageous risk-taking, though ultimately the decision is mine to discern and do what seems best. I hope God is saying to my family, just as the angel said to Joseph, "Do not be afraid to stick with Mary/Mom, for what is transpiring is governed by God's purposes!" That invitation is at the very heart of my Christmas celebration this year.

51 🌿

Is It OK Just to Eat Cookies?

Sunday, December 22, 2013, 2 p.m.

Daughter Judy is baking this afternoon, making little choco-late-cherry dimples and pistachio-cherry shortbread cookies. A friend dropped off pumpkin bread. I know I'm supposed to have lots of protein these days, but I could live on cookies alone.

A few little health observations: "You are getting s-l-e-e-p-y . . ."—all afternoon. I can't complain, though; yesterday I took two naps and then slept seven hours overnight without waking up. That's a record! Today I dragged myself to church early, just to hear and sing a few Christmas carols during 8:15 worship, and I've been half-awake since. Andy says it is time for a walk around the block—can I do it?

I get the hiccups when I take a drink of water. It's the esophagus thing working mischief again.

The radiation burn is breaking down the skin on my left collarbone. Medicated cream three times a day and wound dressing barely keep it in check. The doc might be able to recommend something more healing tomorrow.

Tonight we're going to watch one of our all-time favorite Christmas movies. I have a film lined up for each night this week: *Hook, It's a Wonderful Life, Miracle on 34th Street, The Snowman,* and *White Christmas.* Because it is unwise to plunge into the church crowds on Christmas Eve, I'm saving my Christmas sacred music playlist—and a plate of Judy's cookies—for when the rest of the family goes to church.

52 🌿

Christ Enters My World:
The Gospel of Mark

I CONTINUE TO PUSH BACK against the tide of other topics and preoccupations this week, to ponder the meaning of Christmas for my silent night of cancer. If Christ came into *the* world, is it not reasonable to appreciate that he came into *my* world too? How so?

The gospel of Mark has no obvious birth narrative. Mark's story of Jesus's life begins thirty years later, with the prophetic announcement of his cousin John: "Prepare the way of the Lord" (1:3). We have no Bethlehem scene, no frustrating search for a room, no angels, no shepherds on a magical night. Instead we have a scruffy wild man out by the Jordan River, a prophet of bad diet and humble demeanor who, nevertheless, brings the most important news of all: "The one more powerful than I" is about to crash in on the scene and turn the world upside down.

Mark's action-packed first chapter unfolds the breathless story of the Christ's invasion into public life. The Father's affirmation at Jesus's baptism prepares him for the forty-day wilderness test, after which Jesus enters into the lives of the sick, possessed, busy, feverish, and unclean citizens of Galilee. He correlates his actions to his teaching, and vice versa, so that people can understand that the kingdom of God is being made manifest right in front of them. It is nothing short of an invasion, which is certainly another way of looking at the incarnation. When the power of God breaks in, things happen and old realities fall.

Jesus Christ has been a palpable presence in my life since the summer of 1970—forty-three years ago now. He hasn't had to come crashing in to get my attention since then, though he has been more insistent at some times than others. Suppose you were to get the cancer diagnosis without yet knowing the power of God in your life; it happens to people all the time. Would Jesus's entry into the moment match the force of that diagnosis? For many the kingdom of God is so foreign as to be unrecognizable. Without its stabilizing power, the first feelings After Diagnosis can be overwhelming, numbing, or frightening.

I'm sure first-century Galileans, who knew a lot less than we do about medicine and cure, experienced feelings like these. Many of the people who met Jesus in Galilee were trapped in chronic illness or downtrodden by hopeless circumstances. Their expectations for healing or turnaround might not have been high. Part of Christ's "crashing" is that wonderful jolt of recognition: Here is somebody who can help me.

I can attest that Jesus has helped me. He was there when I got the bad news. He has held me together since. He has lifted his mighty arm to protect me from much of the potential collateral damage from treatment. He has showered me with love from family and friends. I have experienced no trauma because God has been steadily present, deflecting any sense of threat or insecurity.

If in your life you have missed Bethlehem and have not had a kind and gentle introduction to the Savior yet, today is the day to let him invade your reality. Why wait until there is a crisis? Why assume that someday this faith thing will work itself out and you'll suddenly believe in a good God who might help you if you ask? Now would be a very good time to meet Jesus, get familiar with his voice, let his Word inform your reality, and otherwise practice being friends with him. When the Big Challenge hits you (and there will be one), you will already be strong from the inside out, assured of God's power working on your behalf.

The second gospel introduces us to Jesus as a proactive agent of God's grace, willing to have his garment touched, his ankles hugged, and his schedule interrupted. What he brings to our lives is action and courage

in the face of forces that might otherwise do us in. What better response
to this gracious coming than the words of a favorite carol?

> O come, all ye faithful, *joyful* and *triumphant*!
> O come ye, o come ye to Bethlehem.
> Come and behold him, born the King of angels!
> O come let us adore him, Christ the Lord!

53 🖋

Christus Enters My World: The Gospel of Luke

MONDAY, DECEMBER 23, 2013

TODAY WE COME TO THE most beloved version of the Christmas story, the long narrative found in the gospel of Luke. The orderly account of extraordinary events shouts "Miracle! Miracle!" from the beginning of chapter 1 to the end of chapter 2. The details, the characters, the cast of thousands (angels, shepherds, a crowded Bethlehem) surround the essential, sacred truth: God broke into history, conceiving Jesus in Mary's womb, birthing him away from home under difficult circumstances, and working the redemption that would save the world from its sin. From a human perspective, we catch a glimpse of the impossibility of it all, even as we see how God worked in the tiniest details to fulfill his promise of a Messiah.

Two facets from Luke's account reflect how Christ entered my world: he entered *the* world and *my* world by the Holy Spirit and in power.

The Holy Spirit. Luke's gospel is infused with references to the Holy Spirit. All the principal characters of Luke's birth narrative have encounters with the Holy Spirit. The Spirit fills them (John the Baptist, Mary, Elizabeth, Zechariah), informs them (shepherds, Simeon), guides them, and, in particular, is God's agent (for want of a better word) to conceive Jesus within Mary's womb. The reader begins to see that nothing in this story happens by chance but rather is orchestrated and conducted by the mighty hand of God. The resulting music is an exuberant chorus of praise from all who have felt the touch of God.

Power. The touch of God is electrifying and effective. Zechariah is silenced until God proves the truth of his promise. Elizabeth conceives a child in her old age. Lowly Mary is lifted out of obscurity to do the Lord's amazing will. A child is born. The glory of the Lord shines. Angels sing. A star rises. All this power that makes the impossible happen emanates from the one helpless babe lying in the manger. "Nothing is impossible with God" (1:37).

I have not mentioned the Holy Spirit by name in the last few weeks, referring to God mostly in the first and second person of the Trinity. It's time to highlight "the shy member of the Trinity" (Dale Bruner). We understand the Spirit, fully God and distinctly personal, to be the One in Three dwelling in our hearts by faith in Jesus Christ. The apostle Paul did much to enrich our theology of the Holy Spirit. But the "filling of the Holy Spirit" is also, and first, prominent in Luke; the evangelist also speaks of those overshadowed (1:35) and encountered ("come upon" in 2:25) by the Almighty. Along each of their paths, the characters of Luke's nativity story run into the Spirit, who takes over, takes charge, and effects the will of God.

When I tell my story about the out-from-left-field nature of my cancer and the radical right-turn it has required in my life, I feel these events as an overshadowing of the Almighty. To be clear: I do not believe God caused my cancer. In my gut, I feel it as an attack from God's enemy. God, who is never off duty nor taken by surprise at the audacity of his opponent, moved in with the Spirit's power to help me. God's Spirit within me kept me more keenly in touch with God's purposes in this new duty assignment and immediately filled me with a clear sense of calling. BC *and* AD, the life God has given me to lead is a good life, accompanied and overshadowed by a good God who is making all things new.

My experience has also led me to believe in miracles. For years I have had a wood carving that says, "Expect a miracle." I don't know when or where I got it, but there it is right under the light switch above the kitchen counter. If nothing is impossible with God, then my healing is within God's miracle-working capabilities. God the Great Physician is able to turn around a nasty disease. God, who is the Lord and Father of all creation, is able to control errant cells. God, who creates life out of nothing, doesn't require a contribution from me to do his work. God is in the business of doing the life-giving thing, to redeem and create wholeness. God knows enough, sees enough, loves enough, and is good enough to right what is wrong in this world—and in my body. This "reconciling the world to himself" (2 Cor. 5:19) is why he came and why his coming elicits such a chorus of praise from shepherds, peasants, and now me!

54 ✍

Christ in My World and Yours:
The Gospel of John

TUESDAY, DECEMBER 24, 2013, 5 A.M.

I AWOKE AT TWO O'CLOCK this morning, thinking to the point of distraction about the meeting with my surgeon at eleven. I felt not trepidation but excitement and a teacher's love for detailed preparation. And then I remembered the day—Christmas Eve—and my chosen spiritual discipline for the week, to put even a medical consultation in the context of Christ's glorious incarnation.

In the fourth gospel, John presents a unique take on the person and work of Jesus Christ. The beloved disciple, having believed in Christ for decades and staked his life upon the claims Jesus made while walking among us, begins his account by uniting the *Word* concept (a very Greek idea) to the *Messiah* concept (the central Jewish expectation). "And the Word became flesh and lived ["pitched his tent" in the Greek] among us, and we have seen his glory, the glory as of a father's only son, full of grace and truth" (1:14). To John, Jesus Christ is no mere concept but the spittin' image of God in our human experience. For all his "Word" talk, John announces this gospel is anchored in real life. Therefore, we can legitimately ask the same question as before: In what manner has Jesus entered *the* world and *my* world?

What did Jesus Christ bring into the world with him? What is it about his personal character or his attributes that is a particular gift to someone experiencing life's difficulties, be they illness, financial calamity, grief, hunger, relational strain, or discouragement? For many of us, these trials shape our world. But John says Jesus broke through a barrier and entered our world with something that would ultimately overcome it all.

Like the angels in Luke, John announces to the world: Jesus Christ came bringing Life and Light. "What has come into being in him was life, the life was the light of all people. The light shines in the darkness, and the darkness did not overcome it" (1:4–5). The world, trending toward death, was confronted with Life—the power of the one eternal, living God. Jesus would demonstrate the power of this Life at his resurrection, showing the world that the principalities and powers opposed to God were vanquished. Nothing could keep him in the grave. Death could not overcome God's power to live.

The world tripping around in darkness has seen a great light in Jesus Christ. Though God's opponent would like us to believe that the world's situation is hopeless, degraded, murderous, and vile, Jesus has shone a light on the complete picture. His light is purifying, warm, and revealing. It is a challenge to everything that is impure, cold, and deceptive. Darkness cannot extinguish God's light. Jesus proved this by moving into our neighborhood, rolling up his sleeves, and getting to work to bring Life, joy, warmth, and purity into our lives.

I can state with conviction that the application to my situation is "joyful and triumphant." Circumstances are not what they seem. Behind the scene of worldly death and destruction is the Almighty God who desires Life—certainly, spiritual vitality and even now physical endurance—for me. The pressure to believe solely in death outcomes does not come from God. But we can be sure God is at work when we embrace hope, reject fear of death, and live each moment fully and well. I expect to have fun at today's crucial meeting with the doctor, because I have nothing to lose and everything to gain by embracing a *healing* process. Only Jesus Christ, the Word become flesh, can make my experience a positive one.

John's second announcement is that Jesus is the light of all people, including me. I can expect my relationship with him to be characterized by truth-telling, repentance, and integrity. Anything shadowy must flee in the overwhelming presence of God's light. Any voice that speaks lies into my spirit—like "You are not worth all the medical efforts," or "You won't be able to withstand the treatments," or "Who do you think you are, writing about this? Nobody wants to hear from you," or "Be afraid; be very afraid"—is coming straight out of dark corners from a cowering, cowardly, and defeated foe, the Enemy of God and therefore not my friend either.

By rejecting these lies of darkness, I am not espousing a mind-over-matter dynamic. The realities about which I write are not dependent upon my "right thinking" but represent the Light and Life Jesus has brought to the world objectively, whether I believe in them or not. It isn't your belief in what I am writing that will lift you out of your death-and-darkness place; the power of God himself will do that, and in fact has done. The invitation is merely to receive that great Gift on this special day and trust in the One who came to live in your neighborhood to accompany you on your own dangerous journey.

One of my favorite Christmas carols for theological depth and wholehearted proclamation is "Hark! The Herald Angels Sing." The last verse carries it home:

> Hail the heav'n-born Prince of Peace! Hail the
> Sun of Righteousness!
> Light and life to all he brings, ris'n with heal-
> ing in his wings. [Malachi 4:2]
> Mild he lays his glory by, born that [we] no
> more may die!
> Born to raise the sons of earth, born to give
> them second birth.
> Hark! The herald angels sing: "Glory to the
> newborn King!"

55 ✄

Christmas Eve Meeting with the Surgeon

TUESDAY, DECEMBER 24, 2013, 2:30 P.M.

THE WHOLE FAMILY (ANDY, KATY, Doug, Judy, and I) drove to Dr. Straznicka's office, bearing "brain food" (a Christmas cookie platter), discussion chart, and note pad. The nurse ushered us into the conference room in the back of their office space, and soon we heard Dr. Straznicka's clacking heels coming down the hallway. She had studied the CT scan and had the written report in front of her. She looked at the post-it chart on the wall, glanced at her watch (we had thirty minutes scheduled), and off we went. The questions at hand: Has this tumor shrunk sufficiently to make surgery a viable option? Or is continued radiation a better approach?

Before this meeting it looked like definitive radiation (to 60-Gray) made the most sense. However, under the "risk" side, Dr. Straz said the only way to tell whether additional radiation has been completely successful is if the cancer never comes back. If the malignancy were to recur, surgery would no longer be an option, because definitive radiation permanently compromises the healing process of those tissues. I hesitate to cut off future options.

On the plus side for surgery, the good news is that the tumor volume has shrunk by 60 percent. More importantly, it has shrunk in the right direction; there is now space between it and the blood vessels and central structures nearby, making resection possible. The situation will only improve as the lingering effect of radiation continues the shrinkage.

Dr. Straz recommends one more round of chemo before the surgery. "Get the maximum benefit out of continuous treatment, then go in and clean it up surgically." At that time she can eyeball the situation, examine lymph nodes, and remove the entire lung lobe. The best news is that, since I am healthy and fit and my lungs are otherwise in fine shape, I should be able to do everything I did before without compromise. This is not true of many patients, for instance those whose smoking has limited their ability to recover. Also, she believes it might be possible to remove the entire lung lobe by thoracoscopy (the chest equivalent to laparoscopy), requiring only three small incisions and a tiny video camera as a guide. If something sticks or a complication develops, she can enlarge one of the incisions and spread the ribs. I would expect a five-day hospital stay, then six to eight weeks postoperative recovery time. Just in time for hiking season.

Surgery it is! No more radiation.

56 ✍

The First Day of Christmas:
A Baby Wrapped in Cloth

THURSDAY, DECEMBER 26, 2013

A PERFECTLY LOVELY DAY UNFOLDED for the Naegeli family yesterday. We surrounded each other with love, gifts, food, frivolity, and even a little suspense in the annual Christmas treasure hunt Andy instigates. When I needed to sleep, I conked out in my recliner. When I awoke I was amazed that the dishes had been washed, the trash taken out, and card games played.

A recurring gift theme for me was fabric, in the form of soft clothing, headscarves, and cute hats. I am set for life in the scarf department, with several vivid colors and patterns to choose from. Each time I opened a new one, the previous one came off and I wrapped a new turban on my head. The website "Fifty Ways to Tie a Headscarf" entertained us all morning. I have decided to wear my wig only in public among strangers; otherwise, I will express myself with the color and texture of scarves in the next few months.

In light of this celebration of fabric, a detail in Luke's version of the Christmas story intrigues me. When Mary gave birth to Jesus, she "wrapped him in bands of cloth" (2:7). When the angel announced, "It's a boy!" to the shepherds, he said, "Here's the sign: a baby wrapped in bands of cloth . . ." (2:12).

What strikes me is the level of detail, especially of something so common and obvious when it comes to babies. Newborns are always wrapped snugly in some sort of "receiving blanket," presumably to comfort them with womb-like coziness. It should come as no surprise that Jesus's entry into the world of daylight is softened by a swaddle of cloths. So why highlight this seemingly insignificant detail?

First, Jesus was a baby like any other baby. He was treated normally. He "came in the flesh," and he would have suffered cold if he had not been swaddled.

Second, could it be that at the beginning of Jesus's story, Luke is alerting us to the end of his story? Consider the possibility that we are being directed to think about the bands of cloth that wrapped Jesus's dead body after his crucifixion (Luke 23:53)—the same wrapping left in the grave when he rose on Easter morning (Luke 24:12).

It seems to me that those bands of cloth, rough muslin or fine linen, are signals to us of the dynamic purpose of Jesus's human life. If he is to be the Savior, the Messiah, then the full arc of his story is important, from birth through life to death and resurrection. Follow the cloth, and you will follow Jesus's mission: the hem of his garment was the touchstone of healing (Luke 8:44); Lazarus's miracle was celebrated in Christ's command, "Unwrap him!" (John 11:44).

So when I wrap my head in dazzling color in the coming months, I will remember two things: I will remember that Jesus came and was really here in our midst, loved by his mother, swaddled in humanity, and dressed for his mission to me and the world. I will also receive the love that has been wrapped around me. As one gift giver wrote in the card accompanying her cashmere knit hat, "When you wear this, you are wearing a hug from your long-distance family." I love that. By extension, I understand that hug to be from God, too, and plan on passing it along as I am able in the coming months.

57 ✿

The Second Day of Christmas:
A Virgin Deep in Thought

FRIDAY, DECEMBER 27, 2013, 4 A.M.

ONE OF THE DELIGHTFUL SIDE stories to my cancer journey has been getting to know my caregivers. All my doctors (medical oncologist, radiation oncologist, and surgeon) are women with unique and distinguished backgrounds. After this morning I will have seen all three within a week, and each has provided good information to me while staying in close touch with each other. I am comforted to know how well they collaborate and how they have kept me briefed on progress, decision points, and options.

When my family and I met with the surgeon on Tuesday to discuss the next steps, we had to take into account the fact that not only is my surgeon pregnant, her baby is due in less than two weeks! I don't know how this detail slipped past me earlier (although I have seen the surgeon most often in the operating room, when other things were on our minds). It will be her second child, her first being twenty-one months old. We were able to work out the scheduling of my lung surgery and the timing of her baby's arrival. But in the course of the discussion, we two mothers understood each other. It got me to thinking about another woman whose pregnancy rocked her world and had significant implications for others: Mary, the mother of Jesus.

Luke 1:27–38 records Mary's encounter with the angel, who announced to her the impending birth of "the Son of the Most High." Upon hearing the angel's greeting, Luke says, "[Mary] was much perplexed and pondered what sort of greeting this might be."

The young maiden received an out-from-left-field assignment from God with calm curiosity. She first listened to the message Gabriel brought her. Then she asked, "How can this be, since I am a virgin?"—a logical question I could picture myself posing in her shoes. Upon hearing the explanation, Mary said, "OK, I'm in—let it be as you have said." Three steps in a progression of acceptance: pondering, processing, and participating.

When women become pregnant, the process of embracing the new reality begins with a lot of deep pondering. Regardless of how one feels about the turn of events—shocked, happy, fearful, resigned, thankful— there is much to think about. Today's young mothers know within days of suspecting a pregnancy whether they are indeed "with child." Mary, in our story, also knew immediately because the angel told her what was happening. Mary had a full nine months to treasure rich thoughts, uncertainties, and plans, in anticipation of the coming of the Lord. Pregnancy is a time for reflection, for dreaming, for being honest before God.

A pregnancy also requires some planning and processing: When is the baby due? Can I work until the baby comes? Is the baby healthy, and how can I take care of myself to ensure he or she will be okay? What kind of prenatal care will I need? How is my husband coping with all of this? Or, in Mary's case, what will my betrothed (Joseph) think of me now? The feelings overwhelm as a new reality sets in: We are now taking into account the existence of another human being and creating an environment in which the little one can flourish.

There comes a point in pregnancy when a mom is reassured that things are off to a healthy start, and fears abate. Notification is given to family and friends, a new wardrobe is arranged, and preparations are made for baby's arrival. And by the end of nine months, discomforts from heartburn and kicks in the ribs overcome misgivings. All Mom wants to do is give birth.

I have taken a risk here of losing my male readers, with all this talk of a unique female experience. But regardless of our sex, the fact is, every one of us at one time or another receives a new assignment that takes priority over the day-to-day responsibilities we already have. How we handle the duty change depends on our relationship with the one in charge. How well do we embrace a new responsibility that was not our idea? Does it help to see such an opportunity as a manifestation of God's sovereign will?

This whole concept has been put to the test in my new reality: having cancer and shifting my efforts away from a busy professional life to a healing process that could take months, if not years. For you it may be giving attention to a special-needs kid or getting your workplace out of financial trouble. But whatever your new assignment, Mary's example suggests that entering it reflectively asking good questions of God and yielding to God's gracious hand are all part of the healthy Christian life.

58 🌢

A Plan Takes Shape

FRIDAY, DECEMBER 27, 2013, NOON.

TODAY'S APPOINTMENT WITH THE MEDICAL oncologist, Dr. Gigi Chen, was encouraging and decisive. Though my white count is slowly sinking, it is still within normal range. The red count is now officially in "anemic" territory, but not severely. Dr. Chen is amazed at how well I am doing and for this reason is recommending the following course of treatment:

- One round of chemotherapy, starting January 13
- Surgery at least six weeks later, which puts it in late February or early March
- Another round of chemotherapy (fourth total) when post-op recovery is complete

In the meantime, Dr. Chen advises a ten- to fifteen-minute walk outside every day, more, I presume, if I can tolerate it. Fatigue is considered the new normal, due to both radiation and chemo. But exercise is good for body and soul. My brother, who used to work at Los Alamos Labs, is quite impressed with the 4500 rads I have absorbed in radiation—"No wonder you are so tired!" says he who measured his exposure in fractions of single digits. It's a wonder I don't glow in the dark.

59 🌸

The Third Day of Christmas: An Angel Sent to Tell

THE CANCER JOURNEY INVOLVES MANY notifications—exchanges of news, lab results, or even game changers midway through a course of treatment. Most often the messenger is the doctor, or, in my case, one of three doctors representing various disciplines.

The psychology of notification is a fine art. The news one hears can shock, exhilarate, or depress, but rarely just inform. In June of 1998, a hospital nurse called in the middle of the night to tell my father-in-law, "You need to be here." My mother-in-law was being treated for a severe stroke. The complete message would have been, "Your wife has died." The shock of that unexpected news over the phone, however, could have caused an automobile accident and compounded the tragedy of the moment. It was pure grace to summon Dad to the ICU without revealing what had happened until a supportive staff could surround him.

God takes as much care delivering good news as bad; we have ample evidence of this in the gospels' narratives surrounding Jesus's coming. The agent of communication is the angel, appearing several times in Luke 1 and 2, identified as "Gabriel, who stands in the presence of God" (1:19). The overall news he delivers is fantastic: Mary is to give birth to a son who is conceived within her by the Holy Spirit. He will be known as the Son of God and Messiah. The angel continues: others will recognize him as a descendant of King of David's line, and he will do a great work among the people. Wow. This is a lot more information than most mothers, even today, get upon notification of their pregnancy!

But there's more: the angel was sent also to tend to the emotions generated by the news. In Zechariah's case the angel's task was to wake the priest up to the impending miracle that, despite his wife Elizabeth's advanced age, they would be having a baby. Too bad he scoffed and doubted, but this reaction did not thwart God's plan for John (the Baptizer). The angel had to explain the whole process as well as silence Zechariah's objections until the birth occurred. When Zechariah's tongue was loosed at the proper time, it was clear that the nine-month hiatus from talking had done him good; all that came out was praise and thanks to God. But it had taken a while for Zechariah to get there emotionally. God knew, and God tailor made his notifications to Zechariah's needs.

In Mary's case the angel had to consider the possibility of fear. "Be not afraid," Gabriel said, for he was bringing great news, not bad news. It was a good and necessary spin, especially considering that in the short term Mary would be dealing with the stigma of an unwed pregnancy, a difficult third-trimester journey to Bethlehem for the census, and less-than-ideal birthing accommodations, followed by threats from a maniacal Herod against her son. In the long term, what was about to happen would be awesome news, not only for her—a handmaid chosen for special work by God—but also for all of humanity who would be saved from sin by the Son of God that she would bring into the world. We see the fruit of God's gracious tending of her spirit and her emotional health in the Magnificat (1:46–55).

These stories suggest that news that comes from God can be received thankfully, realistically, and confidently. We need not fear what God has to tell us; he is preparing us for what is ahead. The question is whether we are sufficiently in tune with God's Spirit to catch the clues, hear the Word, and otherwise abide in the shalom of life in Christ. Though at times years have passed—many, in some cases—without any special information from God as to what is ahead, God *has* spoken a word into my life at certain key moments. In each case, it was a word that helped me prepare for what was to come or face a reality I had been avoiding. Though it's difficult to explain, such a revelation is accompanied by sweet realism, courage for the day, and God's power to walk the path being paved before me. The thud of bad news has always been paired with the thunder of God's mighty declaration that this, too, can be overcome with his help.

This is why the "bad" news on November 4 that I had cancer sparked no inner drama. The messenger was forthright, factual, and compassionate; she was also committed to helping me and encouraging about the possibilities for treatment. Inside me, God was tending my spirit and stabilizing my reaction. I did not experience any fear or trauma (and still haven't), because God has convinced me that I am protected and safe. God's Word has real teeth at a time like this: "Even though I walk through the darkest valley, I fear no evil; for you are with me; your rod and your staff—they comfort me" (Ps. 23:4).

On this third day of Christmas, it would serve us well to remember that God can and does tell us what we need to know when we need to know it. Even bad news—from a human point of view—remains navigable on God's map. We are probably not strong enough to handle life's twists and crashes on our own, but God is, and he has promised courage. "Do not fear, for I am with you. Do not be afraid, for I am your God. I will strengthen you; I will help you. I will uphold you with my victorious right hand" (Isa. 41:10).

At such a time God speaks his message of life and hope into our lives, because no circumstance can diminish God's ability to carry us through it. "Nothing is impossible with God" (Luke 1:37), and "the zeal of the Lord will accomplish it!" (Isa. 9:7).

60 ✒

An Active Day: Just an Experiment

SUNDAY, DECEMBER 29, 2013, 3:45 A.M.

THIS PAST WEEK MY FATIGUE was more pronounced. "Just as it should be," said the doctor on Friday, since I am now slightly anemic, on top of the effects of all that radiation.

The gathered family has been trying to catch all the hot movies this week, and Friday night they went to see *Hunger Games: Catching Fire* without me—mostly because, at twelve dollars a pop, I didn't want to fall asleep in the theater.

But when they left, I started a slow putter that gathered into a perfect storm of activity: I cleaned up the kitchen, made chocolate/marzipan truffles, and prepared a quiche for the next morning's brunch. Then I went to bed and read a book until they got home. Who knows where the energy for all that came from? But I had fun.

Then yesterday Andy had the brilliant idea to take a low-risk excursion over to Richmond and the WWII Home Front National Historical Park and the Rosie the Riveter Museum. Ninety-two-year-old Park Ranger Betty Soskins was giving a talk at 2:00 p.m. It was so good to get out there by the Bay on a gorgeous day, with pelicans and seagulls flying low overhead and the smell of sea salt invigorating the soul. We ambled through the exhibit, watched a movie about Japanese internment camps, and then enjoyed the presentation by Ranger Betty.

I almost threw up from the exertion, but it was worth it.

61 ✍

The Fourth Day of Christmas:
A Marriage Morphs into Parenthood

SUNDAY, DECEMBER 29, 2013, 7:30 A.M.

AS WE CONTINUE OUR CELEBRATION of Christmastide, carrying with us the realities of human existence like cancer and other soul-burdens, I don't want to miss a detail in Luke's account related to Zechariah and Elizabeth. This priestly couple had enjoyed—or endured, depending on one's point of view—a childless marriage for decades. It had been long enough for Elizabeth to absorb the shameful label "barren." In her culture the inability to bear children was viewed as a sign that God had withheld blessing, that something was wrong with them, and that their family line would soon be obliterated.

This circumstance did not stand in the way of Zechariah's conducting his priestly duty at the temple. And it's a good thing because Zechariah meets an angel in the sanctuary of the Lord. The priest is terrified by Gabriel's appearance (1:12). Conditioned, I imagine, by years of failure and disappointment, he becomes a bit belligerent when told his wife will bear him a son (1:18). Unhappy with Zechariah's response, Gabriel asserts his authority: "I stand in the presence of God, and I have been sent to speak to you to bring this good news" (1:19). Zechariah is struck dumb while the angel explains what is to happen.

Having lost his voice, all Zechariah can do as he emerges from the sanctuary is to pantomime something. Did he try to mime "angel," as if he were playing charades? We do know that when his temple term was up, he went back to his home, where "his wife conceived" (1:24). Connect the dots here: despite his skepticism, despite the history, despite a sense of hopelessness and shame that had crept into their relationship, despite their age, Zechariah and Elizabeth came together and conceived a child. Now that was an act of faith! Nothing is impossible with God.

When God brings a new reality into our lives—something new or out of left field like my cancer diagnosis—he invites us to live into the new reality as an act of faith. My new duty assignment AD (After Diagnosis) calls me to enter fully into the cancer reality, as much as I hate to relinquish the illusion of health or lay aside my professional life. The purpose of entering reality fully is to fulfill my new calling and to be fully present to God, who is ready to meet me in this place. Someday, presumably like Zechariah and Elizabeth, I might be able to say that this life is what I would have chosen. As it is, this life is what has been given, and I choose to receive it graciously in order to be the person God has called me to be. That new discipleship entails cooperating with treatments, enduring the discomforts joyfully, resting in cancer fatigue, and otherwise going with a much slower flow than I am used to. No longer am I a foot-loose-and-fancy-free agent but a duty-bound patient with a new health history, for the purpose of bearing new fruit yet unseen.

God has given each of us a unique path to walk and a life to lead, though we do not always understand God's purposes. Unforeseen circumstances become God's invitation to bear new fruit in a new, unanticipated way. A response of joy and thankfulness makes us available to God, ready to offer that fruit in his service.

62 🖋

The Fifth Day of Christmas:
A Decree and a Prophecy Meet

MONDAY, DECEMBER 30, 2013

WE AMERICANS CHERISH FREEDOM SO dearly that we sometimes resist the inclinations of big government. A national ID card, for instance, cannot get traction. Every tenth year we hear about folks who desire not to be counted in the census. The unveiling of the NSA's data-tracking mission has made people even more paranoid about their personal information. The registration form at every new medical office asks me to provide my Social Security number, which I decline to give. I think more than rugged individualism accounts for this; people desire to retain control over their lives and don't think more government intrusion is going to help them.

Today's meditation revolves around an earlier government intrusion at the direction of Roman Emperor Caesar Augustus. He issued a decree around 4 BC that everyone in his world was to be registered. The presumption is that the emperor was getting ready to extract new taxes and needed to identify his tax base. In Israel the decree was organized by ancestral tribe: each head of household was required to go back to his ancestral home village for the census.

Joseph, now engaged to Mary, who was heavy with child, lived in Nazareth but identified home as Bethlehem. Hence the uncomfortable journey south, a distance of about eighty miles, probably accomplished in a caravan moving about twenty miles a day. But at the end of the road, Joseph and Mary were on their own, looking for lodging in a city bursting at the seams.

Meanwhile, those who knew their Scriptures knew the prophecy that the Messiah would come from Bethlehem:

> But you, O Bethlehem of Ephrathah,
> who are one of the little clans of Judah,
> from you shall come forth for me
> one who is to rule in Israel,
> whose origin is from of old,
> from ancient days. (Micah 5:2)

We have no indication from Luke's text that Joseph and Mary had connected the dots and seen their migration to Bethlehem as anything but fulfillment of a civic duty. And yet, in retrospect, we can't help but see the connection that, years later, slowly dawned on Jesus's contemporaries: "Has not the Scripture said that the Messiah is descended from David and comes from Bethlehem, the village where David lived?" (John 7:42). God has used the movements of history, the whims of despots, and even geography to accomplish his will. In this case, what would move this couple, at such an inconvenient time, to travel to a little town and give birth in a strange place? It certainly wasn't their idea. It took an act of a godless emperor to make it happen.

When we become frustrated with circumstances that seem out of our control, we can consider how God has moved us into new places we never would have traveled otherwise. If God had a mission for me in this cancer world, he would have to get me here; and he did. I am free, to a certain degree, to make choices in this new place. But being here is not optional. I cannot protest that God has intruded in my life. May the Lord continue to help me see my existence as a "living sacrifice" offered in worship to my Creator and Lord every single day!

63 ✦

The Sixth Day of Christmas: Shepherds Roused from Sleep

TUESDAY, DECEMBER 31, 2013

YESTERDAY WAS THE FIRST DAY without any cancer treatments, medical appointments, or lab tests. I hardly knew what to do with myself. If it hadn't been for my daughter's presence, I would have been lonesome, bored, and unimaginative. Even with her company, I spent most of the day ensconced in my recliner under the residual effects of radiation and chemo—that deep fatigue hard to describe, but oh, so concrete in experience. After a nap I spent another hour mustering the will and the strength to get up for my obligatory fifteen-minute walk around the neighborhood.

On this sixth day of Christmas, we look to the shepherds who were in the hill country surrounding Bethlehem on the night of Jesus's birth. They roughed it every night, sleeping outdoors with their flocks and keeping a watchful eye out for predators. Not known for their refinement or for wealth, the shepherds represented the unimaginative, lonesome, perhaps bored underclass of people. The Bible has some notable shepherds in its cast: Joseph son of Jacob, Moses, David, Amos, and Jesus. Isaiah used the image of shepherding to describe the responsibility of the Jewish leaders of Israel, whose inattentiveness led the chosen down a path to destruction. God seemed to like shepherds, but the rest of society didn't have a high opinion of them. It's a dirty job, but somebody has to do it.

So, our Bethlehem-area shepherds are out in the open air doing their job, no doubt sleepy in the middle of the night. Nobody would notice or even care about them. But because of their unknowing proximity to Mary, Joseph, and Jesus upon his birth, they had the experience of a lifetime. An angel appeared before them, accompanied by "the glory of the Lord," which we interpret as blinding light. The shepherds were terrified, perhaps wondering if they were in the middle of a vivid dream. The angel—laughing in great joy, maybe—told them, "Hey, no need to be afraid! I'm bringing some great news: It's a boy! And not just any new baby, but a Savior, the Messiah! You should go and take a look!"

After consulting with each another—for these were men with responsibilities—the shepherds decided they should hurry over to Bethlehem for a look-see. They were so overtaken by the importance and urgency of the moment that their regular duties faded into the background, and their fatigue was completely overcome by excitement. They found Jesus and his earthly parents right where the angel said. Something made a big impression upon them because they told everybody they could about the visit.

The middle of the night, or the middle of cancer fatigue, is a time of low expectation for most of us. We're not expecting an angelic visit or even a phone call announcing the birth of an awaited baby. Let's face it: through draggy days we are glued to our recliners, invisible to most people, slow on the uptake physically and spiritually. While all may be quiet and still in our own family rooms, somewhere close by Jesus is at work shepherding a wayward people, making an appearance in an otherwise hopeless situation, or moving someone to give testimony to Jesus's presence and power.

Do we need an angel to tell us what God is doing? No, we need only eyes to see and ears to hear. We're talking about the spiritual gift of discernment, the God-given ability to pick up on what is happening spiritually and to act wisely to God's glory.

How long has it been since you became aware of something God was doing in your neighborhood, your workplace, or among your family members? Have you been so sleepy that you have missed the signs? Take stock: do you know enough about those around you to pick up on God's activity in their lives? An indication of God's protection? A spark of God's creativity? A changed attitude toward the Christian faith? An act of loving compassion toward "the least of these"?

Why would you want to know that these sorts of things are happening? Because that is where Jesus is being born in our midst! In those places of love, compassion, service, or sacrifice, our Lord is making kingdom headway on earth as in heaven. What a great privilege it is to recognize and marvel at the work God is doing. You don't want to miss the wonders because of inertia.

> How long will you lie there, O lazybones?
>   When will you rise from your sleep?
> A little sleep, a little slumber,
>   a little folding of the hands to rest,
> and poverty will come upon you like a robber,
>   and want, like an armed warrior. (Prov. 6:9–11)

64 ✍

The Seventh Day of Christmas:
A King Blinded by Pride

WEDNESDAY, JANUARY 1, 2014

IT IS A NAEGELI FAMILY tradition on New Year's Eve to pass the hours between dinner and midnight by watching the 1995 A&E version of *Pride and Prejudice*. It never ceases to delight and vex, and we recite our favorite lines in the course of the five-hour-fifteen-minute presentation. If we plan it just right, the wedding bells begin to ring right on the stroke of midnight.

Jane Austen's novel, as suggested by the title, revolves around the predispositions of the two main characters. Mr. Darcy (Colin Firth) is a sulking, prideful man who is fixated on class and position; Miss Elizabeth Bennett (Jennifer Ehle) forms prejudicial opinions of people based on mere scraps of information. How their pride and prejudice unfold provides terrific psychological suspense and a great love story. The attentive watcher (or reader) is prompted to self-examine for those same traits. To help us, we have another character in the Christmas story.

Matthew 2 opens with King Herod's getting wind of rumors that a rival king has been born. Matthew says Herod was frightened (2:3), which is interesting, considering the power he wielded to frighten everyone else. But the prideful king, known for his paranoia, was fixated on retaining his position. So he hatched a plan to kill his rival—a demonstration of pure pride. We also see his prejudice: with little information, Herod concluded that the baby born in Bethlehem must not survive infancy. He saw Jesus's birth as a threat to his temporal power because he knew no other application for the word "king"; he showed no sign of recognizing the kingdom of God.

One's own perception of self and the world is the starting point of pride and prejudice. Pride assigns greater worth to oneself than to others, and prejudice veils an accurate view of others. A person afflicted with these character traits cannot receive God's message easily, and Herod is a glaring example of where that can lead.

Helmut Thielicke, in *The Evangelical Faith*,[7] describes the difference between a Cartesian worldview (René Descartes, "I think, therefore I am") and a non-Cartesian worldview, in which God's thought and action are sovereign over all. It is extremely important that we trade our limited view of self and the world for God's view. For example, the former defines God according to one's own experience rather than by God's revelation of himself.

C.S. Lewis captured this idea in *The Screwtape Letters*. Screwtape instructs the junior devil Wormwood to divert the human's prayers away from God to a human image of God: "For if [the human] ever comes to make the distinction, if ever he consciously directs his prayers 'not to what I think You [God] are but *to what You know Yourself to be*,' our situation is, for the moment, desperate."[8]

If, with the Lord's help, we can see the world and ourselves through God's eyes, we are in a position to accept the reality of our sin, receive its remedy, live the transformed life, and walk in the light of God's presence. But if we remain stuck in our limited, self-centered perception, creating an imitation universe we supposedly can define and control, we will not be dealing with spiritual reality at all.

Seeing the necessity to change, how do we turn our own pride and prejudice around? We begin by acknowledging our self-centered view

---

[7] *The Evangelical Faith* by Helmut Thielicke, 2 volumes (Grand Rapids, MI: Wm. B. Eerdmans, 1974).

[8] *The Screwtape Letters* by C. S. Lewis (New York: HarperCollins, 2001), letter 4, "The Painful Subject of Prayer" (emphasis added).

and our propensity to define God in our own terms. Then we ask God to help us know him as he really is. It was a conscious act for me, as my faith was being formed, to put my pride and prejudice on the shelf in order for God to make himself known to me. Early in my Christian walk, for instance, I was introduced to Christian fellowship beyond the parochialism of my Catholic upbringing. God spoke to me through study of his Word, from Genesis to Revelation, in the company of believers I could not "see" before the Spirit pointed them out. As God's self-revelation boisterously intruded upon me, God not only revealed his character but also redefined mine. Embracing all the graces and benefits of knowing Jesus as my Savior and Lord, I am under construction, as God removes the props of pride and prejudice from my life.

65 🖋

The Eighth Day of Christmas:
The Multitude of Angels

MY WORLD HAS BECOME SMALLER since my diagnosis. Before I got sick, I was traveling to Kenya and Uganda on vacation. Now a twenty-minute walk around the block is a major field trip. Anyone I see must come to me, since public places pose a significant risk to my suppressed immune system during flu season. One is lulled into believing that reality is very small and even quiet. But the eighth day of Christmas carries a reminder of the noisy and boisterous reality surrounding the God of the universe.

The shepherds operated in a small world and had a single task. Granted, at night the heavenly canopy was theirs to gaze upon and enjoy. And it wouldn't surprise me if shepherds gathered when the day's work was done for storytelling and perhaps a little playacting. But they were an uneducated and uncouth underclass. They were not recreational travelers, scholars, or philosophers. Their world was small and, for the most part, peaceful.

So that night when the first angel appeared to the shepherds to tell them about Jesus's birth, they got their first glimpse of glory. That experience alone would have been enough to rock their world. But what happened next was absolutely mind-boggling:

> And suddenly there was with the angel a multitude of the
> heavenly host, praising God and saying, "Glory to God in
> the highest heaven, and on earth peace among those whom
> he favors!" (Matt. 2:13f)

All of a sudden, a *multitude* of angels appeared! Heaven opened up
and blessings poured out upon the shepherds through this vision of the
heavenly host united in song, giving glory to God. The shepherds would
never be the same.

Angels appear throughout the Bible, singly, in pairs and trios, and
sometimes even in multitudes. According to the writer of Hebrews, their
purpose is to maintain perpetual worship of God and to be available
for divine service (1:4–14). That service takes many forms: announcing
God's good news and judgment, protecting vulnerable people, celebrating conversions, and ministering through trial and temptation. They are
spirits and therefore immortal, but they are not gods. They operate in
the presence of God, regardless of the particular task to which they are
assigned.

When the shepherds' senses were overwhelmed with the chorus of
a multitude of angels, it was as if a curtain parted to reveal what is ordinarily going on out of our sight. Heaven leaked its tuneful blessing that
night, and the shepherds' world immediately expanded.

I have never had a moment in which I felt heaven leaked into my
world quite so literally. But the fact that a chorus of angels has not per-
formed specifically for me bothers me not at all. I am content knowing
a concert awaits me when I make the journey from this life to the next
(a *long* time from now, I pray). I also know without a doubt that such
a vision is possible and that the angels are constantly engaged in this
amazing musical happening, all for the glory of God and the witness to
his power and might.

Nevertheless, I pray once in a while for a leak from heaven. Along
with the apostle Paul, "I consider that the sufferings of this present time
are not worth comparing with the glory about to be revealed to us" (Rom.
8:18). At times of deepest discouragement, it is a comfort to ask Jesus for
just a moment of heavenly eyesight, for just a tiny leak of his glory to

keep me going. But reading about it in the Scriptures is enough for now. I am content, knowing the world I experience is but a tiny fraction of God's far greater glory.

66 ✑

The Ninth Day of Christmas:
A Sign Seals a Covenant

FRIDAY, JANUARY 3, 2014

I HAVE DISCOVERED IN MY cancer journey that milestones must be celebrated with some kind of ritual, both for fun and to mark progress and acknowledge what is happening. For instance, the night before I started chemo, we enjoyed fellowship with friends—among them several Presbyterian elders—who gather monthly for "family dinner." They laid hands on me and prayed for the success of my treatment, according to James 5:13–15. Last night I celebrated the end of round two and its aftereffects by going to a movie, my first in months. Moments like this must be marked, and I will continue the practice until cancer is a thing of the past for me. When *that* day arrives, we're throwing one heck of a party, I promise you.

In Luke's account of Jesus's nativity, the angel points to an important Jewish milestone: on the eighth day after his birth, Jesus would be circumcised and given a name. Luke's report is short and sweet: "After eight days had passed, it was time to circumcise the child; and he was called Jesus, the name given by the angel before he was conceived in the womb" (Luke 2:21).

Circumcision was ordained by God as a sign of his covenant with the chosen people, Israel (Gen. 17:12). A particular scar marked those (males) who were dedicated to the Lord and welcomed into the household of faith. The mark was permanent and personal, individualizing the commitment of a people to God. So why would Jesus, God's Son, submit to this ritual?

It would be important to Jesus's mission to be identified as part of the chosen people, as circumcision signifies. Naming the child was also part of the ritual. Some say waiting eight days before naming was recognition that the child might not survive birth; after the first perilous eight days, it was okay to embrace and welcome the baby. I am more apt to take the Lord's command at face value, which would put circumcision in a faith-expressing rather than utilitarian context. The naming of a child identifies him as a child of the covenant, set apart from the world unto the Lord in faith and service. This idea, by the way, is carried forward into the Christian baptism of male and female infants, according to the Catholic, Orthodox, and Protestant traditions.

Later Jesus would receive John's water baptism at the Jordan River. At that time Jesus would be identified publicly as God's Son ("with whom I am well pleased") and propelled into ministry (Luke 3:21f; 4:1–19). This practice reiterates the idea from the Old Testament that the chosen have been given a commission. God told Abraham he would be "blessed to be a blessing to all the nations" (Gen. 12:1–3). The name *Yeshua* ("God saves") indicates Jesus's calling as Messiah and Savior.

Similarly, when we are named "Christian" at baptism and confess our faith, we are marked with the seal of the Holy Spirit, a "circumcision of the heart" (Rom. 2:29). In addition, it is important for Christian adults to mark important moments in our faith development—dates of our choosing, not dictated by Law.

This might include what the church has called confirmation, but even birthdays will do, or days in the church year, or reception as a new member of a congregation. Other holy days on your personal Christian calendar might include occasions when you made a new faith commitment in service or ministry (like ordination) or the birth of your child, a commitment to faithful Christian parenting. These moments carry all the way to our deaths, when we celebrate the resurrection of Jesus Christ and his faithfulness in our lives.

The need for ritual to mark realities includes the Catholic sacrament of the sick—anointing with oil, laying on of hands, and prayer for those who suffer illness. I fully appreciate that lovely rite now that I am sick and in need of progress markers. I look forward to the next family dinner which will occur the night before round three of chemo begins January 13.

67 ✿

The Tenth Day of Christmas:
Two Old Saints Made Happy

SATURDAY, JANUARY 4, 2014

EVERY ONCE IN A WHILE, especially at night, a thought crosses my mind that perhaps I am living the last year or two of my life. I try not to think about this too much, not because I am in denial about the dangers of my disease, but because it gets me in "fear of missing out" mode. It causes me to think about my "bucket list," a term coined by a 2007 movie of that name. Two hospital roommates bust out of a cancer treatment center to embark upon a road trip, during which they do the things they've wanted to do their entire lives.

The bucket list is not a new idea. Forty days after Jesus's birth and about a month after his circumcision, Jesus and his parents went to the temple in Jerusalem to bring an offering. While there they happened upon an old man named Simeon. He was not a priest, but he was "righteous and devout, looking forward to the consolation of Israel" (Luke 2:22–25). Simeon's one life goal was to see the Lord's Messiah, and this was the day for that aspiration to be fulfilled. When Joseph and Mary brought Jesus into the temple, Simeon saw them and scooped the baby into his arms. He recognized the One instantly and proclaimed in the *Nunc Dimittis* the presence of God's salvation, "a light for revelation to the Gentiles and for glory to Israel." Wow. The moment he had been waiting a lifetime to experience.

Simeon had prophetic gifts and uttered some disturbing words about the baby's growing up to be a stumbling block to Israel and a deep sorrow. Luke writes that Simeon also understood Jesus's impact would be global, not limited to Israel—that God's salvation is intended for Gentiles as well as Jews.

Later the prophetess Anna joined Simeon. An eighty-four-year-old widow, she was a daily visitor to the temple for fasting and prayer. When she saw Jesus, she too praised God and exclaimed that he was "the redemption of Israel."

For both those old saints, Jesus's visit to the temple made their day and fulfilled their life's goal, the last item on their bucket list. Their eyes had been fixed on God for a very long time, and they were now rewarded, seeing God's great plan for salvation.

It's fun to think about: What are those things I've always wanted to see or do? I have never been back to Michigan where I was born. I would like to drive across the United States, just to experience its vastness. And a climb up Half Dome in Yosemite still beckons. For years I have said, "I would like to learn how to play the oboe," but I have taken no concrete steps in that direction and probably never will. I want to live long enough to see my daughters settle in their niches in life and to hug grandchildren someday.

"Thinking with the end in mind," as Stephen Covey advised in *Seven Habits of Highly Effective People*,[9] what would I wish to do, and what steps can I take now in that direction? Would anything on that list be spiritual in nature? How I wish that God would reveal to me his cosmic plan for salvation, or even that he would visit me in some special way. I hope that God, who has begun a good work in me, will complete it (Phil. 1:6). I would like to die well, having remained faithful to my Savior until the end of my life.

I think it is the thing we hope for that defines us. If we hope for riches, our striving will define us. If we hope for survival, our struggle

[9] Stephen R. Covey, *The 7 Habits of Highly Effective People: Powerful Lessons in Personal Change* (New York: Fireside/Simon & Schuster, 1989), 95–144.

will define us. If we hope for revenge, anger will define us. If we hope for the Lord's salvation, our humility will define us. As time passes and our hopes distill within us, we become more and more like what we hope for. Our hopes become our essence, and that essence expresses itself in our attitudes, aspirations, and actions later in life.

Many years ago Presbyterian pastor Ben Patterson wrote in an article that as his aging aunt got older, she became sweeter and sweeter. She had always been a dear soul, but Patterson saw that as she neared her death, she was "reducing to her essence." By the same token, a gentleman of his parish, who had been a thorn in Patterson's side for years, also reduced to his essence as a complainer. The question is, What trajectory am I on? What do I pin my hopes on? What do I dwell on? Those are the things that will define me later in life. Would it not be good to have our eyes fixed on Jesus, the author and perfecter of our faith (Heb. 12:2), so that Christlikeness becomes our essence? That goal summarizes my bucket list, and I trust that what Jesus has begun in me he will complete as promised (Phil. 1:6).

68 ✍

The Eleventh Day of Christmas: Wise Men Curious about That Star

A COUPLE WEEKS AGO I had a big decision to make about my cancer treatment: whether to continue radiation to a definitive level and forgo surgery, or to consider radiation complete at its current preoperative level and undergo lung surgery. I put together a chart to help in the decision-making process. I started with a few known facts, but the rest was speculation based on studies and research data. Ultimately, it was up to me to decide; I wished there were more entries in the Known Facts column to guide me.

When it's dark, literally or figuratively, it is difficult to see ahead, much less navigate. Life involves a lot of guesswork, so God is generous with his offer: "Hey, if you realize you don't have enough wisdom, ask me, and I will provide plenty of it" (Jas. 1:15). At times I don't even realize that there is a need or that God is providing an answer to a question I haven't asked yet.

I think the magi were facing the answer to an unasked question as they looked at the heavens around the time of Jesus's birth. The stargazers were professionals from Persia or Saudi Arabia who studied the heavens for omens and clues to life. They might have been astrologers, but they were not "kings." The Scriptures say they were "magi" (or "wise men") who noticed something extraordinary in the sky and derived meaning from it. (A supernova? A confluence of two planets? Many interesting studies have speculated about what could have produced a persistent "bright star.") What the magi saw moved them to action because, by their interpretation, the bright object in the sky was leading them to something they needed to find. How they came up with the name "king of the Jews" I do not know, but that fact led them logically to Israel's capital, Jerusalem (Matt. 2:1–6). The natural phenomenon got them close to the action but not quite to a full revelation, which would come when the Jewish teachers they consulted showed them the Scriptures.

God's faithfulness provided a means for Gentiles to find Jesus in an unexpected place. God used language those magi could understand—astronomical phenomena—to bring them into the Nativity scene. They followed God's leading and found a new King worthy of their worship.

I'm not a stargazer myself, but God has intruded upon my life in other ways. My cancer diagnosis has been accompanied by God-sightings, and he is giving me a certain amount of wisdom to discern his leadership through this valley. Throughout the history of God's people, Abraham, Moses, David, Solomon, and many others experienced God's direct leading. I am convinced God wants to lead us through our own wilderness experiences.

I may never have enough entries in the Known Facts column to quiet my questions about the future. But I pray that I will recognize "the star" at the right moments and be willing to go where God leads me.

69 ✒

Weight Gain

I AM REGAINING STRENGTH BETWEEN chemo rounds. The next round be-gins in a week, so I'm trying to walk more every day and make up for lost time. Yesterday I walked 1.2 miles on flat city streets—the farthest I've gone in months, and it didn't exhaust me at all. So today I conquered a four hundred-foot climb in our local Open Space with Rocky Balboa enthusiasm.

My weight has shot up. Some of this can be attributed to unbridled holiday eating, but not all of it. Ten pounds in four weeks? Cisplatin can cause this, and it's generally not good; it could indicate that I am not drinking enough water for kidney health. So today I am keeping closer tabs on my water consumption. The doctor also suggests that the steroid Decadron could be fostering weight gain: "But don't worry; when you're done with chemo, that weight will just drop off."

Though I felt up to it, I decided not to go to church today because of the germs freely exchanged there. Now is not the time to get sick. I was surrounded by coughers all through the holidays and didn't catch anything, for which I am very grateful.

Yesterday I received a phone call from our friends Steve and Alene in Kenya. Supportive communications have come from Africa, Argentina, Mexico, and Japan. Praise God for the many churches that include me on their prayer lists. Though in the short term I have settled into a medical routine, I don't want to get used to having cancer, because some day I'm not going to have it anymore. Bolstered by those healing prayers across the miles, I expect to be fully alive for the calling God gives me then!

70 ✒

The Twelfth Day of Christmas:
Magi Bearing Gifts

Monday, January 6, 2014

THIS TWELFTH DAY OF CHRISTMASTIDE is a special day on my personal calendar. Eighteen years ago on this date, my father died suddenly of a cerebral hemorrhage. At the time I processed his swift departure from this life with gratitude for his own epiphany. For all the fears we carry about death, the Christian belief that we shall see Jesus when we die is supremely comforting. We so often hear the words "So-and-so is in a better place now," and this well-meaning cliché is not untrue. But what is really a balm to the soul is to know that our Christ-believing loved ones are with a better person.

We can only guess what was in the minds of the magi as they set out on their great journey from known to unknown. Is our destination a better place than our homeland? Is this king a better person than our own rulers? The wise men made their trek west, following the star, to Jerusalem, where they met with King Herod. This was a logical stopover for the strangers since they were looking for "the king of the Jews." But when they got to Jerusalem, it was clear they were in the wrong place, talking to the wrong person. They were looking for another; with the clues they gleaned from Scriptures shared by teachers of the Jewish Law, they realized this and moved on to where Jesus was.

> They set out; and there, ahead of them, went the star that they
> had seen at its rising, until it stopped over the place where the
> child was. When they saw that the star had stopped, they
> were overwhelmed with joy. On entering the house, they saw
> the child with Mary his mother; and they knelt down and
> paid him homage. Then, opening their treasure chests, they
> offered him gifts of gold, frankincense, and myrrh. (Matt.
> 2:9–11)

We're accustomed to our crèche scenes that depict shepherds and
wise men present at the same time. But it did not happen that way. To
understand the chronology of events, we must weave Luke's and Matthew's accounts together.

Assuming the star did not appear until the night of Jesus's birth, the
magi would not have begun their journey until then. Herod's murder of
the "innocents" (all babies born within the last two years) suggests that
it took a long time for the magi to arrive in Jerusalem. Herod pointed
them to Bethlehem, according to his knowledge of the Old Testament
prophecies. But Matthew says the star "stopped over the place where the
child was . . . [O]n coming to the house, they saw [him]." There was
no "house" in Bethlehem, so there is a possibility that this wonderful
encounter took place at the family home another eighty miles north, in
Nazareth.

The important thing is this: when the wise men found the child
Jesus, they knew they had arrived. When they saw the child with his
mother, their first instinct and reaction was to bow down and worship
him. Even when directed toward a king, such humility is an amazing
acknowledgment.

And with their worship came very valuable gifts: gold (a precious
metal), incense (a spice), and myrrh (a balm). Not the most practical gifts
for a toddler but symbols of the esteem and power ascribed to the child.
And we cannot miss the connection with the end of the story: myrrh
and spices were used to anoint Jesus's body upon his death by crucifixion
(John 19:39).

When we gather for worship, the magi remind us, it is not good to come empty handed. It is a sign of our esteem for Jesus Christ and recognition of his power that we bring a gift. This may be a tithe, a donation of food for the poor, or some other tangible offering. When we come bearing gifts for God, we are making a statement and offering our hearts in fully engaged worship.

> What can I give Him, poor as I am?
> If I were a shepherd I would bring Him a lamb.
> If I were a wise man, I would do my part.
> But what can I give Him? I will give Him my heart.

We bring our heart to worship as our relational gift. This too is what the magi brought when they bowed down to worship Jesus, the infant king. Far outshining the material offerings were their heart-gifts of loyalty and allegiance.

When my father left this life and moved to heaven, he by necessity arrived empty-handed, but not empty-hearted. Right alongside the magi he now participates in the ongoing symphony of praise directed to the One who sits on the throne of grace and majesty.

EPIPHANY

71 🌿

Spurring One Another On

THURSDAY, JANUARY 9, 2014

C ANCER TREATMENT VARIES, DEPENDING ON the type and stage of one's particular disease. The protocols tend to be repetitive and cyclical. In my case, chemotherapy runs on a four-week cycle: one week plus one day "on" and the remainder of the four weeks "off," while I recover from its rigors. By the time week four rolls around, I am feeling pretty good—almost normal. This is one of those weeks, and I am getting a lot of things done around the house as a result.

Round 3 of chemo begins on Monday. Since I can plan on feeling sleepy and tired the first and second week of the cycle, someone is with me during that time. But on a week like this one, I need no help, so while Andy is at work it's just me here at home. I can get out to run a few errands or meet someone for lunch, but generally I am alone without feeling lonely.

But I also am not having much face-to-face interaction with people. I realized last night, as I attended my first small group study among church friends in months, how much I thrive in an interactive Christian environment. I was thoroughly engaged, entertained by the others' stories, and enjoying the book we were discussing. My mind was stimulated, and I was reminded how much the teaching/learning dynamic fuels my soul. I have missed teaching this fall and interacting with students, either at the seminary or in my church family. The past two full weeks by myself, without any medical appointments, has had its own side effect: a bit of withering on the vine for lack of stimulating conversation.

This issue is not unique to me. Mothers of young children often come to church expressing delight at having an adult conversation. Elderly church members who become homebound are often deeply grateful for the soul tending that accompanies a friendly visit. Human interaction keeps us sharp and alert.

The writer of Hebrews speaks to what I feel:

> And let us consider how to provoke one another to love and good deeds, not neglecting to meet together, as is the habit of some, but encouraging one another, and all the more as you see the Day approaching. (Heb. 10:24f)

Prior to this passage in Hebrews the writer makes a case for adopting habits that enable believers to persevere through difficulties. These habits include coming to God in prayer, remembering Jesus's acts of redemption and forgiveness, and holding fast to the hope we profess. These disciplines can be done privately, in times of personal devotion. But the fourth habit of Hebrews 10:24, meeting together to encourage love and good deeds, must be done in Christian fellowship.

What about people like me who both need and want this "spurring" but for one reason or another cannot get out to fellowship with others? That's a call for the church family to bring the fellowship to us: to stay in touch, to share the sacrament of Communion, to converse about the faith, or even to sit with us in silent companionship. People need this, and historically Christians have been very good at providing it.

People like me need more than comfort while navigating a challenge. We need encouragement to live out our discipleship right here, right now, and not squander the opportunity for spiritual growth and meaningful ministry that exists even from the chemo chair.

Years ago I was teaching a class on Christian discipleship, and an elderly person raised her hand and said, "You know, I get what you are teaching us, but my strength and ability to get out are so limited, I don't think there's anything I can really do now in ministry." She said this with some resignation, even sadness, in her voice. You should have seen the other fellowship members gather around this lovely lady to "spur her on to love and good deeds." They gently asked her a few questions about her lifestyle and limitations, and then they said, "But Mabel, we know how much you love to pray. What if you became the point-person for the church's prayer chain? You have a tender listening ear. Our intercessors would love to have your help." It was a beautiful thing to help her see the value of what she *could* do!

So I am adopting a personal challenge, on these chemo-"off" weeks, to have spiritually oriented conversation with someone at least every other day. I need the prod in my side to keep me involved and learning. You teach me or let me teach you, but let's get together to encourage one another in faith and ministry!

72 ✒

Everything Is on Course

FRIDAY, JANUARY 10, 2014

TODAY WAS MY CHECKUP WITH the nurse practitioner prior to starting round three of chemo on Monday. Blood counts (white, red, platelets) are all sinking slowly, but this is par for the course. She does not characterize me as seriously immunosuppressed but advises some caution during flu season. Going out in public is okay as long as it isn't a packed-like-sardines situation (like BART at rush hour). With this encouragement, Andy and I will enjoy a dinner out and go for a drive.

I certainly feel well enough for some outside activity. Yesterday, for a little upper-body workout, I pruned our fig tree. I've been walking at least a mile every day. All this goes out the window on Monday, of course, but that too means the meds are working. I continue to praise God for my progress so far without some of the losses I expected (like appetite and taste buds). Yes, I feel a bit like a blimp with this eleven pounds of extra weight, but by summer I hope that will be gone. Meanwhile, it's a good thing I still have some "fat clothes" in the closet.

Today in the cancer center waiting room, I encountered *three* friends also there for consultation, treatment, or shots. It was like old-home week, comparing notes, encouraging one another, giving thanks to God for progress and blessing. I got home a half hour late because of the conversations.

73 🍃

Suppressed Immunities

A S MY BLOOD COUNTS SINK lower, my immunity to "normal" disease and viruses diminishes. To avoid picking up the flu or a head cold, I keep my hands washed and don't touch my face. I finally got a flu shot yesterday. Avoiding sickness requires vigilance and a little paranoia, but it is possible.

Translate that to the strenuous efforts people make to avoid being exposed to the gospel. A few people in my life are so resistant to the gospel of Jesus Christ, it's as if they have masked and gloved up in order to keep any part of the message from reaching them. One got a little bit of church in childhood—enough to inoculate him from the real thing in adulthood. If the conversation ever drifts in the direction of Christian faith, resistance surges, the discussion veers, and the subject changes.

Such folks keep their distance from books and ideas that lift up the Christian faith. They certainly wouldn't be caught dead in an actual church. It is as if they have developed a serious allergy; the slightest exposure to anything faith-related makes them sneeze and gasp for air.

This religious allergy requires believers to find ways to get people in touch with the Savior that do not evoke such violent responses. Sometimes that means being very oblique in the approach, witnessing through actions and not words, and joining them in common causes in which we can work together. However, if this notion makes *us* allergic to *sharing* the gospel, then something really terrible has happened. The question is, *How* do we share the gospel in a gracious, nonthreatening way?

We are called to live our lives as Christ followers and reflect thoughtfully on what we are learning along the way. We do not have to shy away from conversing specifically about that; but we can use vocabulary familiar to our friends rather than buzz words that only have meaning within an isolated church context. We can view our present experience as life on a journey toward Jesus and share pictures of the scenery along the way. In other words, we need to overcome our own religious allergies and begin deciphering for our friends what the Word of God means to us in a particular situation and how that Word directs our response.

In my small group this week, a gentleman indicated that what kept him from being open on the subject of faith was not any adverse reaction from the not-yet-believer but fear that he might get a question he couldn't answer! Such an admission tickles my heart, because "there's an app for that." The more a person learns, the more at ease that person can be in respectful conversation with someone whose views are different or undeveloped.

Above all, I believe that God's Spirit can empower us for the gentle but persuasive work of the kingdom.

74 ✒

The Law of Love as We Share
Our Faith

Tuesday, January 14, 2014, 6:30 a.m.

I've been considering how to tell people about Jesus, the one who is carrying me through my cancer journey. I am getting over my reticence regarding the gospel with the religiously allergic people in my social circle. But one situation offers an exception.

Some of the people we have close relationships with are family members who are no longer of the same mind religiously. They are less likely to sing out of the same hymnal or maintain the same spiritual and religious vocabulary. Some may even have chucked the faith altogether.

My family of origin and my next-generation family represent the entire spectrum of belief, from professed atheism to strong Christian orthodoxy, from liberal to conservative Christianity, from committed Roman Catholic to ordained Presbyterian to nondenominational. Let's just say the potential for fireworks at Thanksgiving is enormous.

I continue to live my life for Christ as best I can and manage the current challenge of lung cancer, *and* I have a burning passion for giving a nonambiguous witness to the gospel of Jesus Christ. Even so, I know that a conversation with certain family members about the Bible, Christian faith, or their personal spiritual journey is off the table. We've had those conversations before, and they have made themselves clear, their lives reflect their decisions and values, and they are living out their various commitments as consistently as they know how. If Jesus were in my shoes and relating with my family, what would he be doing in response to these apparent closed doors?

He would love each and every one of my family members. Just love them. He would find ways to relate to them on their turf. He would ask the question internally, "How does [so-and-so] receive love, and what of that can I give to convey my affection for this unique creation of God?" I may think it is love to advance an uninvited theological argument, because everybody needs the Savior, right? That is certainly true, but insisting on it constantly is like hammering our beloved on the head. An intermediate step—and perhaps the only step—is for me to love them with consistent kindness, respect, active listening, generosity, and good humor. Just as we love our little children in such a way that they can eventually grasp the nature of their heavenly Father's love for them, so we love all those with whom we have a family relationship.

What I am learning is that our love for our siblings, parents, or children becomes conditional if we are constantly pushing them for a decision for Christ. What Jesus is saying to me is this: You're past the point of convincing them of anything. Just love them. Don't wait until they make a decision that you approve of or that conforms to your standards of belief and practice. Love them today; embrace them as they are. Keep praying for them, but do not let Christian conversion be the condition for your love. Today, affirm them in those qualities that encourage you, give you joy, and that make sense in their current situation. Rejoice when they rejoice, weep when they weep. Privately you may grieve over some of their choices, but that is Jesus's burden to bear, and he will help you translate that mourning into gladness.

This is how I understand the law of love as it plays out in my family relationships. In all things, our motivation is gratitude for the unconditional love God has poured into us over a lifetime, not waiting until we were presentable or converted. He has loved us from the beginning of life and held out great hope for us. With that security and hope, we can do the same for those around us.

75 🌿

Back in the Saddle Again

TUESDAY, JANUARY 14, 2014 7:30 P.M.

WE GOT OFF TO A good start on round three yesterday, with a four-and-a half-hour infusion of five different drugs. Nurse Judi checked my medical record and discovered the doctor had decided to stay with the full dose of the steroid Decadron rather than risk any possible nausea. I'll do the best I can with this weight gain for now.

In the meantime, I praise God that the worst potential side effects are not showing up, giving me more freedom to focus on my calling of writing and encouraging others. So that's what I'm trying to concentrate on.

Yesterday I received a lovely note from a group of friends who miss seeing me at church. Last week the men's Bible study from the first church I served sent a card of encouragement signed by all the men present. It is prayer and support like this that holds me up and holds me together for the Lord's service.

LENT

76 ✍

Ashes to Ashes

WEDNESDAY, JANUARY 15, 2014

THE CHURCH YEAR MOVES TOWARD the penitential season called Lent, which begins on Ash Wednesday. The service on that day usually includes "the imposition of ashes," which takes on new meaning for me this year. The minister marks my forehead with ash in the form of a cross, saying, "Remember, woman, you are dust, and to dust you shall return." These ritual words confront my mortality.

I have not encountered the diagnosis of cancer without thinking about where it might lead. I'm talking about death, this great enemy of humanity, and now of mine. Death's shadow has been lurking in my mind since before Christmas, when I batted it away in favor of "Joy to the World." It comes out now not because my thoughts are turning morbid or because I am depressed, but because it is time. Lung cancer is inviting me to stare the great enemy in the face.

In a sense, though, my foe is not God's foe. According to the psalmist, "Precious in the sight of the LORD is the death of his faithful ones" (Ps. 116:15). Solomon, too, noted, "The day of death [is better] than the day of birth" (Eccl. 7:1). Jarring as these statements might seem to a person in the throes of dying, they simply point to God's perspective on our transition from this life to the next: precious and better.

The story of our mortality began in the garden when Adam and Eve fell from grace (Gen. 3). The ultimate consequence of their rebellion against God was to be ejected from Paradise, thereby losing access to the Tree of Life (3:24). That was when we humans lost our immortality; without the Tree of Life our bodies were now subject to physical death. As horrible as this seems to us, God removed us from the garden in the hope that we would eventually be reconciled with him. God did not want us eating from the Tree of Life while we were in this new sinful condition, thus perpetuating our alienation forever. God could not allow us to close the door permanently. By ejecting us from the garden, God gave all people the opportunity to be reintroduced to their Creator, even while undergoing the stresses, diseases, and toil of everyday life. The end of this life is physical death, after which we may, if we have embraced Christ, enter into eternal life free of crying, mourning, pain, and death (Rev. 21:4). Even God is looking forward to that, for our sakes.

Living this side of the garden gives us plenty to think about and yearn for. The apostle Paul himself lived in two worlds, a thought that comforted me as I dealt with the unexpected death of my good friend Henry Greene. Paul was a citizen of both earth and heaven, even as he pursued his preaching mission. He believed that to live a while longer allowed his ministry to continue, while to die was to regain immortality. Either way, Paul said, I win (Phil. 1:21–26). Paul had a clear vision of life in eternity and looked forward to it. But he also knew that leaving (that is, dying) would cut his earthly ministry short. The timing of the transition was up to God, but it was not to be feared.

The reality of death and fear of it hides in the back of our minds and motivates us in one way or another. Whether we fear or embrace the inevitability of our physical demise, it is going to happen sometime in our future. Lent is a good time to explore what that means and open the doors to spiritual growth.

77 ✒

Grieving in the Process of Dying

THURSDAY, JANUARY 16, 2014

IN THE 1960S, A SWISS psychiatrist working at the University of Chicago Hospital observed a progression of emotions experienced by dying patients. Elisabeth Kübler-Ross, MD, conducted seminars in which the dying were interviewed regarding their feelings about death. Although her research outraged the medical establishment, Dr. Kübler-Ross identified five stages of grief. In subsequent decades, her theory was overly applied to include the experience of many losses—death of a spouse, divorce, job termination, house fire—but recent corrective studies have differentiated between those and the primary focus of Kübler-Ross's original observations.[10]

As the possibility of my death looms, I can see some reactions that follow Kübler-Ross's pattern.

Stage 1: Denial, or "No, not me." Immediately before my diagnosis, the possibility of cancer flitted across my mind. I pressed it out of the way because *I am strong. There has been no cancer in my family. It can't happen*

---

[10] Elisabeth Kübler-Ross, *On Death and Dying: What the Dying Have to Teach Doctors, Nurses, Clergy and Their Own Families* (New York: Scribner & Sons, 1969). For a critique of Kübler-Ross's theory, see Christopher Hall, "Beyond Kübler-Ross: Recent Developments in Our Understanding of Death and Bereavement," *InPsych 2011*, Vol. 33, Issue 6 (December 2011), accessed at https://www.psychology.org.au/for-members/publications/inpsych/2011/dec/Beyond-Kubler-Ross-Recent-developments-in-our-und.

to me. After Dr. Straznicka gave me the news and I followed up with Dr. Chen, I avoided any approach of life-threat as painfully as a wallflower avoids eye contact at the school dance.

Shock and disbelief are natural reactions to such news; they are the body's means of protection from a severe, overwhelming reality. In the face of such an intruder, we slam the door, until we are able to open it a crack and let the news seep in. Denial might take overt forms of disbelief or protest. Or we might isolate ourselves from particular reminders or realities. I once knew a family man who, after a diagnosis of cancer, holed up in his bedroom, refusing to talk to anyone about it for months. We each need denial in varying degrees and for varying lengths of time, to ease our absorption of the truth. Eventually, we are able to acknowledge what has happened.

Stage 2: Anger, or "Why me?" Whittled down to its essence, the second stage of grief is outrage. A life-threatening diagnosis, by definition, takes something of mine away. I want life to go on. I want to keep working. And I really want to feel self-reliant, dignified, and healthy. When something we want is denied, we get angry. My reaction to the cancer diagnosis: "But I've avoided bad air my whole life and I've never smoked! So why should I get lung cancer?" After my father's sudden death, my mom was angry that she then had to do all the driving. These days I get ticked off that I am *not* permitted to drive.

An observer might be tempted to judge bursts of anger harshly. Anger is, after all, one of the seven deadly sins. But the apostle Paul suggests another way of looking at this powerful emotion: "In your anger do not sin" (Eph. 4:26). What if we saw anger as a pointer to the deeper work that is necessary to cope with our impending death? The challenge is to handle our anger respectfully, yet without sinning. This deeper work can start out looking ugly, as a loved one rails at the healthy, sues a caregiver, or shakes a fist at God.

Stage 3: Bargaining, or "Why now?" When my death is expected and anger is in play, I might feel that asking nicely can prevent or at least postpone the inevitable. According to Kübler-Ross, the patient makes promises of good behavior in exchange for a guaranteed life extension or relief from pain. Martin Luther's famous oath on a dangerously stormy night was a bargain of desperation: "If you get me out of this storm alive, I will go into the priesthood."

My bargaining has taken the form of fastidious compliance with diagnostic and cancer treatment regimens. "If I show up for every appointment, take every treatment, and drink enough fluids, then Lord, won't you count me in that slim margin of lung cancer survivors? I would really like to see my grandchildren born." Bargaining may last a brief period or many months and years, with a prolonged illness. But bargaining is sustainable only to a point. Then the next stage of grief looms.

Stage 4: Depression, or "Yes, me." Everything has been tried, every veil pulled down, every topic avoided, every person blamed, every promise made, and still imminent loss looms. The reality of what has happened or is happening can no longer be denied. Depression sets in. We slump in our chair, powerless to reverse what is now inevitable. I acknowledge that I have not experienced serious depression in my own struggle against cancer.

Nevertheless, there are things I miss. It made me sad not to have enough physical strength to go to Henry's memorial service. It depresses me that I am unable to muster the energy for lovemaking, but worse, that even the most gentle touch of my beloved feels bruising, even though it is not. Though real to me, these points of sadness pale in comparison with the experience of a fellow patient. She has the same kind of cancer I do and is undergoing the same treatment regimen. But her tumor didn't shrink, like mine did. Hers continued to grow. As her surgeon said, "This will not end well."

Depression paves the way to acceptance. In its dark valley, the world shrinks and the focus of attention narrows to deal with a growing sense of frailty. The dying often desire to disengage from unnecessary distractions, to limit visits and give energy only to those most important. When their loved one withdraws and enters a period of silence, family members often perceive this as either rejection or defeat. But letting go of everything and everyone who has ever been close to you is the inner work of preparation for death.

Stage 5: Acceptance, or "It's OK now." A quiet peace, a serenity, characterizes the final stage of grief. More than an intellectual justification, this kind of acceptance is experienced deeply, at the emotional level. One yields to the forces at work and embraces them wholly, without a fight or fear.

This is different from resignation. Think of a teenager who, when grounded and denied use of the car, stomps out, yelling, "OK, *fine!*" There's plenty of fight left in that statement of resignation. In contrast, acceptance is characterized by a sense of quiet victory and confidence. I have accepted my diagnosis and loss of health, though death feels distant enough I don't have to accept its inevitability just yet.

In real life the five stages of grief usually progress in a less tidy fashion than I have depicted. Many people move through them in fits and starts, sometimes circling back to a previous stage for a time, until it can be abandoned completely. The painful process of loss and dying requires patience, not only of those experiencing it directly but also of those observing and accompanying them on the journey. Knowing how denial, anger, bargaining, and depression can express themselves has helped me be a more compassionate pastor and a patient more tolerant of the feelings that rise up within me.

78 ✐

Denying Death Doesn't Make Life Better

Friday, January 17, 2014

In 1973 Ernest Becker published a Pulitzer Prize–winning book call *The Denial of Death*.[11] I am finding it more accessible than ever, given my current health situation. His thesis is that all humans have in common a fear of death and that controlling this anxiety is the single most powerful motivator of human behavior. This fear is so terrifying that people "conspire to keep it unconscious" and replace it with conscious, persistent efforts to make themselves immortal or heroic, as a way of transcending death.

Drawing on Christian philosopher Kierkegaard, Becker depicts a primal inner struggle.

It all started in the garden. God created human beings out of the earth, on the same day he fashioned all the animals. Human beings are creatures with bodies, bodies that—after the fall in Genesis 3—must be tended, maintained, treated, fought with, and ultimately dismissed to death. But for humans, the sixth day of creation also included God's deep breathing into our souls to bring us alive as spiritual beings, aware of our relationship with God, who gives life and meaning to our creaturely existence. Integrated as we are in body/spirit, we do everything we can to

[11] Ernest Becker, *The Denial of Death* (New York: Free Press/Simon & Schuster, 1973).

repress the impact of our mortality. Do we want to die? Heck, no! The thought of our annihilation is so outrageous and insulting that we spend our lives avoiding it.

This avoidance can take many forms, all under the heading of "becoming the hero." The dark side expresses itself in dominance, narcissism, and intimidation—whatever it takes to feel oneself the superior overcomer. Becker was no optimist on this score and believed that oppression and war are rooted in the insatiable drive for survival—means to deny one's susceptibility to death.

The light side of the equation represses fear of death by making life meaningful and securing for oneself an indispensable role. Meaning is derived from usefulness and altruism and even "the ultimate sacrifice." Practitioners of this art become superheroes at making lemonade out of lemons. But the root cause is the same: We'll do anything to push back into our subconscious the knowledge that even a heroic life shall pass. King Solomon, who himself had everything and a very good life during Israel's heyday, wrote Ecclesiastes toward the end of his success, concluding that it was all for naught: "I saw all the deeds that are done under the sun; and see, all is vanity and a chasing after wind" (Eccl. 1:14).

The great quest of human beings, and now myself, is this: How can I hold the paradox of both sides of my nature, creaturely and transcendent? Is my faith and confidence expressed in my journal really a diabolical denial of reality, or is it an honest attempt to keep doom and hope in realistic balance? It is hard to grapple with the limitations of my body leading unto death, because I haven't been required to deal with my demise in such concrete terms. In the present grappling, my desire to leave a meaningful legacy through the writing of this book (as one example) cries out to the world, "Don't forget me! Admire me! See, I will never die!"

But our faith offers a different perspective. Seeing myself as God does can help me face my death with more joy and courage than a finished book could ever provide. The apostle Paul, who had invested a lot in being the perfect Jew, a zealous Pharisee out to obliterate the early Christian movement, instead discovered that any strength (or heroism) he had was nothing compared to knowing and promoting the primacy of Jesus Christ the Lord (Phil. 3:4–11). To live for Christ is to serve *him* and *his* purposes, to lift up *his* memory and abide as God's child, empowered by the Holy Spirit to represent *him* in the world. This is a strong antidote to a fear of death, and it carried Paul through deep troubles.

It's no wonder we invest a significant effort in denying death. When our invincibility is challenged, we get angry. We try to work out an alternative plan that results in our survival. But ultimately, "resistance is futile." We are all going to die. Denying this does not make life better.

Accepting death enables us to embrace life all the way to the fulfillment of our story. Counting on eternal life is not a denial of death; it assigns meaning to it. I would rather live with hope in the afterlife than see life as a meaningless dead end. C. S. Lewis captured the hope of all Christians in *The Silver Chair,* when Puddleglum awakens to the witch's lie that the Under World is all there is:

> Suppose we have only dreamed, or made up, all those things—trees and grass and sun and moon and stars and Aslan himself. Then all I can say is that, in that case, the made-up things seem a good deal more important than the real ones. Suppose this black pit of a kingdom of yours is the only world. Well, it strikes me as a pretty poor one. That's why I'm going to stand by the play world. I'm on Aslan's side even if there isn't any Aslan to lead it. I'm going to live as like a Narnian as I can even if there isn't any Narnia.[12]

As a person who loves God and believes in the resurrection of Jesus Christ, my personal hope for immortality is not hypothetical. It is grounded in the amazing scriptural accounts of Jesus, God's Son and Savior of the world, who died a real death, was placed in a real grave, and rolled a real stone away from the grave to emerge risen and really alive. Not only did this happen to him, he promised that we who believe in him would also have eternal life: "I am the resurrection and the life. Those who believe in me, even though they die, will live, and everyone who lives and believes in me will never die" (John 11:25f).

"Even though they die." Yes. "Yet shall they live." Amen.

For this reason, I choose to live like a Narnian.

---

[12] C. S. Lewis, *The Silver Chair* (New York: HarperCollins, 1953, 1981), 12.197.

79 ✇

Death Is a Transition

WHY IS IT SO HARD to face death? When we are young, vigorous, and healthy, death seems irrelevant. But then something happens: a friend dies suddenly, or we note the effects of advancing age, or we encounter a long, life-threatening illness.

All of a sudden, we are not talking hypothetically. I could die of this disease, and I am not ready. But circumstances force me to entertain the possibility that I won't be around. What then?

The first thing I think is, *Darn! I haven't finished the Ahwahnee quilt I designed for our bed.*

And there's that pile of unsorted stuff in my office, saved as evidence of my life and the fruit of my ministry.

Do I really have to go before I get a chance to climb Half Dome? And what about my dear husband and kids . . . can they get along without me? Is there any unfinished business to be dealt with before I go?

These are the thoughts of a perfectionist, a pipe dreamer, an attention seeker, a hoarder, a controller, a doer. Lurking under all those façades is a woman who needs love in the form of safety, security, and, ultimately, salvation. Can that woman—can I—overcome an aversion to the unknown and face the fear of losing the comfortable known?

I am not in such pain or agony to long for death. Infirmity has not rendered me useless. I still have contributions to make in this world. My presence is meaningful and helpful to a few people. And yet, my time may be coming. Is there any way that I can welcome death?

Welcoming may be a stretch, but perhaps accepting death is possible. My faith in the risen Jesus enables me to trust that physical death is not the last word on my existence. I possess an essence, a soul that is distinctly mine, that will live forever. Jesus tells me I will make a transition from this life to a new life. I leave to God some important unfinished business—his business—involving the whole world. When, finally, Christ declares history fulfilled and God's enemies defeated, then eternal life will assign to me a new, cancer-free, energetic body with which to worship and serve God.

I shall be safe. I shall be secure. And I shall be saved.

I shall survive death.

80 ✑

From This Life to the Next

SUNDAY, JANUARY 19, 2014

I<small>T'S THE QUESTION EVERY PARENT</small> dreads: "Mom, where do we go when we die?"

I used to think that when a person died, he or she immediately entered the realm of eternity, because with God there is no time. N. T. Wright's *Surprised by Hope* has caused me to reexamine that view, if for no other reason than this: God has operated within the framework of time ever since he created the world in six days. God is certainly not limited to the time dimension, but his son, Jesus, did enter the world at a particular moment, to become fully present within our time-space limitations (Phil. 2:5ff). Is there something "future" for God? No, everything is present to him. But the Bible recounts for us God's actions within time, unfolding over millennia, even while he dwells in eternity. Let's hang on to that idea as we ponder what happens to us when our time on earth is finished.

In passing from this life to the next, we relinquish a unique but flawed tent, in the words of the apostle Paul, and we take up a new dwelling in God's benevolent presence, for a time (2 Cor. 5:1–4). According to Wright, our entry into eternal life happens in stages; eternity itself—existence outside the time dimension—does not start until after Jesus returns in glory to judge the living and the dead. In other words, life immediately after death still involves waiting in real time. Mind you, we are waiting in paradise, but the culmination of God's cosmic history is yet to come.[13]

This period of waiting is not to be seen as punitive or even purifying—ideas that are attached to the concept of purgatory. Rather, according to Wright, it is an interim existence in a place—really, a *condition*—of conscious but restful abiding in the presence of God.[14]

A Presbyterian pastor once answered the question, How do we pass from this life to the next? with a helpful analogy:

> A little boy, full of life and energy, played and played after dinner until he wound himself down. He curled up on the couch in the family room and fell asleep. At his regular bedtime, his father tenderly carried him, still asleep, from the family room to his bedroom, so that when he awoke the next morning, he was in his own room tucked into his own bed.

Our passage through physical death is like this transition from one room to another: we fall asleep here (our bodies die), and we awake in paradise, alive to Christ in the room prepared for us, as he promised. From a pastoral perspective, I can think of nothing more reassuring than this: "that my only comfort, in life and in death, is that I belong—body and soul—not to myself but to my faithful Savior, Jesus Christ" (Heidelberg Catechism, Q1).

When I am carried through death into that rest, I will experience freedom from cancer, hay fever, pain and suffering, and whatever else ails. In fact, I look forward to basking in the presence of our Creator in paradise while history is completed and Jesus Christ declares his final victory over death itself.

This paradise is not to be seen as the *final* resting place, or "heaven," because that all unfolds after the judgment (Rev. 20) and the joining of the new heaven and the new earth (Rev. 21:1–5). And what a glorious day that will be, when God's people get to enjoy and manage all that has

---

[13] N. T. Wright, *Surprised by Hope: Rethinking Heaven, the Resurrection, and the Mission of the Church* (New York: HarperOne/HarperCollins, 2008), Chapter 10.

[14] Wright, *Surprised by Hope*, Chapter 11.

been made new, reclaimed from the throes of death, disease, mourning, and difficulty. This life *after* life after death is what we will have been waiting for: the place of eternity where there is no need for sun or moon to mark the days, because the Lord's glory is all the light we will ever need (Rev. 22:3–5).

Comforted by the reality of eternal life, I can accept death, my death. It's the dying I am not looking forward to.

81 ✑

Deep Breathing Hurts

MONDAY, JANUARY 20, 2014

AS THE WEEKEND PROCEEDS, MY malaise has also progressed. No one thing is overwhelmingly bad, but a bunch of little things add up. I decided today to cut some fabric for my quilt, but after thirty minutes I was exhausted and took to my chair again.

I think what is happening goes back to something I didn't pay much attention to last Thursday. I had my monthly check-in with the radiation oncologist, whose job is to alert me to possible side effects still in the offing. The interesting thing about radiation is that those effects can accumulate for weeks after the treatments are done. She mentioned the probability that I would experience some inflammation at the site of the tumor, even to the point of causing a new cough. The inflammation will eventually resolve itself, but it can cause some discomfort in the meantime.

Yesterday I realized it hurts to breathe, almost like I pulled a muscle, except that the pain is located inside, where the tumor is. A dull ache discourages me from taking large, deep breaths. Inflammation can also be the source of this generic not-well feeling. So I'll keep an eye on it and certainly be alert to fever. I remind myself that fatigue means progress, so I choose to thank God with joy and patience through this stage.

82 ✐

Prepare to Die—Part 1

AN INTERESTING ARTICLE APPEARED IN Sunday's newspaper, titled "Coffee, Cake & Grave Conversation." It described Death Café, a hosted conversation about death and grief in Santa Cruz (one among many in California).[15] The group's purpose is to formalize discussions "to help ease the anxiety around death and dying." The intended benefit appeared to be both spiritual and practical, as people share and learn about various burial options, celebratory rituals, and advance directives. It reminded me of a series of adult classes we used to have at church, On Death and Dying, in which participants would plan their own funerals, write their obituaries, consider a Five Wishes document, and sign advanced directives, all from a faith perspective. The public Death Café discussions portray spiritual answers as completely personal and therefore not definitive. They do not offer anything more than an information-is-power message while they prepare participants in practical ways for what is to come.

There is a lot to be de-mystified about cancer, and information on that topic, to some degree, is power. Knowing this has motivated me to chronicle my experience in detail for the benefit of others. Engaged as I am in *thinking* about death, *practical* matters are easy to postpone. The

---

[15] Jessica Yadegaran, "Death Café: Coffee, Cake & Grave Conversation," *Contra Costa Times,* January 15, 2014.

death café exercise recommends concrete end-of-life planning as one way to break through the barrier of denial.

Death itself remains an elusive mystery, because we can only talk about the process of dying prior to the event. Once we're dead, we can no longer share our experiences. As a friend so eloquently insisted a couple days ago, death is not the scary thing, it is what happens between now and then—the dying process—that is outrageous and rude and, yes, frightening. Nobody wants to anticipate pain and suffering or indignity, if those experiences are part of one's dying process. Yet this pre-death phase—while we live—is the only realm in which we have at least a bit of control because the matter is taken out of our hands at death's door.

Keeping the end in mind, let's work backward from what we know. We cannot deny that we all will die. I am going to die, and so are you. However, we do not know the way or the means by which this will occur. What must develop within us to enable us to accept the inevitable? And how would that change the way we live in the meantime?

Since the final stage of grief is acceptance, that place of emotional and spiritual repose, each of us would do well to consider what sort of person we must become in order to accept our eventual death. Dallas Willard, in *Renovation of the Heart,* offers the insight that inner transformation is the first step toward outward change.[16] What sort of person is able to die in serenity and joy? What qualities must constitute our most essential being for this to happen? Let's consider at least three things that will be required of us at the moment of our death: resigning, residing, and retiring. Will we be ready to meet this challenge?

Resigning. Turning in our papers, so to speak; withdrawing from the job of living. Pulling out and ceasing work. Declaring we have worked enough and stopping the fight.

Residing. Resting in the fruit of our labor and the depth of God's grace. Abiding in an estate that has been prepared just for us. Declaring ourselves content, satisfied. Basking in the benefits of personal knowledge of our Creator, Redeemer, and Sustainer.

Retiring. Turning in one lifestyle for another completely different

---

[16] Dallas Willard, *Renovation of the Heart: Putting on the Character of Christ* (Colorado Springs, CO: NavPress, 2002), 22–3.

endeavor. Yielding to a new reality, leaving one life behind and embracing new, eternal life in Christ. Allowing my world to shrink enough to concentrate on dying, yet opening my heart to embrace eternity's wonder.

Every single one of us has this faith-challenge ahead. Will we be prepared to let go? Will we have enough to hold us together through the valley of the shadow of death? Will Jesus be enough for us as we face the perplexing questions that dying raises? Will our faith be shaken, or will it be strengthened by the dying process? Will talking about it help? Is information enough power to get us through the ordeal? Or is our power found in another source? Since I am going to die, what can I do to be ready for it? It is, once again, a call to discipleship. Christian disciples slowly develop answers to these questions as they practice trusting the Savior.

83 ✐

Prepare to Die—Part 2

WEDNESDAY, JANUARY 22, 2014

A PARISHIONER FACED HER IMPENDING cancer death by requesting pastoral visits, during which she addressed some concerns about her spiritual condition. She confided that her husband, unable to empathize, was not a conversation partner for her. During our visits, he stoically polished his car and did not respond to friendly greetings. Their different emotional approaches to her dying suggested to me that people need help—long before death is on the horizon—to work through the feelings that later will surface in the stages of grief.

If I observe that I tend to deny unpleasant realities, then practice at facing difficult truth now will help me meet dying later. By meeting smaller problems realistically and practicing the presence of God through life's challenges, we lay the groundwork for confidence even in the face of our demise. Death is difficult and inevitable, but ultimately we will transcend it.

The anger phase of grief can be anticipated and practiced by learning how to deal with everyday anger without sinning (Eph. 4:26). We acknowledge its trigger. We hold appropriate outrage while letting go of the need to punish. We forgive God and people who have frustrated us. Whatever we do, we do not freeze in anger, but do the inner work to release it.

If I anticipate I might strike deals with God (along the lines of "just let me see my kids graduate from high school," or, "anything but cancer," or, "please take me first, not my husband"), now is a good time to have a Job-like sit-down and assess whether the God of the universe strikes deals with mere mortals of so little standing. (Recall Job 38, where God challenges Job's credentials to question the Almighty's purposes.) When the time comes, there might be prayer requests and special favors to ask of God to ease the way, but the cosmic issue of God's authority over my life will have been settled beforehand.

If I am prone to depression, part of death preparation involves getting help to identify the source or cause of deep sadness and learn how to manage it. In my lifetime I have experienced two periods of depression, several years apart. In each case, I learned something significant about myself, about God's faithfulness, and about getting help. Someday, as I approach my death, I may sink into an emotional black hole, but at least I know it is a place where God can meet me tenderly.

The time of our death is the moment of complete and utter surrender to God. We resign our position as a mortal inhabiting this earth. We reside in the sufficiency of God to carry us into eternal life. We retire one life and embrace a new one. This is the final earthly act of our soul, to relinquish all claims to ourselves and stop asserting control, striving, and rebelling. Yes, we give up. There is no shame in that. Remember, "How precious in God's sight is the death of his saints" (Ps. 116:15).

I can't imagine myself being able to do that then if I am unable or unwilling to surrender to God now. This is why Christian discipleship is a critical element in our preparing to die. Learning how to surrender to God now in much smaller things will make the passage from this life to the next much easier when the stakes are cosmic.

So where are the opportunities to practice surrendering our lives to God? Everywhere and every day! When I am oblivious to the work God is trying to do in me, I can ask his Spirit to open my heart to the Word of life so I can learn what God is trying to teach me. When anger flares, I can submit my sense of entitlement to God's will. When I am trying to make deals with God but there's an "out of order" sign on the divine vending machine I have installed, I can remember that God is no machine at all but a loving father. When I sink into sadness over circumstances I cannot control, I am invited to cling to the hope I have found in Jesus Christ.

My pastor friend Rick Carter sent a note a few days ago, summarizing an article by Jackson Carroll called, "The Continuing Conversion of the Pastor: A Call to Renewal." Rick writes:

> After acknowledging some of the reasons why giving ourselves rest from our work is so hard to do, Carroll turns to an obvious reality. At some point in each day, we give up and go to sleep. "Regardless of that resistance to rest, at some point we are forced to quit; we must naturally lie down, give up. We daily practice our death—the final letting go of all."
>
> I found his turn of phrase arresting and thought-provoking. I would guess that very few people view their going to sleep as practicing their death, but what if they did? Our daily relinquishing of ourselves to God as we close our eyes could become a valuable spiritual practice.
>
> Every generation before ours thought about mortality all the time. They taught it to their children. "Now I lay me down to sleep . . . If I should die before I wake . . ." Our generation is moving further away from the contemplation of death, to our detriment. Jackson Carroll reminds us that our daily rhythm of sleeping and waking can be, if we let it, one way to stay rooted in reality, and to daily practice entrusting ourselves to God.

Surrendering to God is part of the daily, abiding life of Christian discipleship. When we fall short, Jesus listens, teaches, forgives, and sets our steps in a new direction. We slowly get used to the idea that Jesus is Lord of all and Shepherd of our souls. And that he can be trusted. Knowing he can be trusted with our living and our dying prepares us to say goodbye to this world in anticipation of the next.

84 ✒

Turnaround to a Full "Work Day"

AFTER A LOUSY WEEKEND, YESTERDAY I woke up early feeling much, much better. I began making some phone calls to the East Coast and by day's end had spent most of the day on the phone getting some nonprofit work accomplished and feeling fully alive and cancer free. My next-door neighbor, Barbara, sat with me, but there wasn't much for her to do on my behalf. While she got a lot of knitting done, I was off to the races. I even had energy left to go to my evening small group Bible study.

This disease is so mysterious and unpredictable. I feel fine today, so I am none the worse for wear. I take the turnaround as a gift. Maybe beefing up my potassium intake helped. Maybe the steroids are still working their positive results. Maybe the Lord is healing me. In any case, I celebrate good days and tolerate bad days and feel carried through both. But yesterday's activity reinforced my desire to be well and to get back to normal life. I think I am on the way.

Meanwhile, I am awaiting word on the exact date of my surgery, tracking a couple of bills through the insurance maze, and otherwise managing my case. This management should get easier, because I have no medical appointments and no treatment for a while. We're in the surgery-preparation phase now, and my goal is to stay healthy—avoid the flu and viruses going around—and get strong.

85 ⬟

Prepare to Die—Part 3

THURSDAY, JANUARY 23, 2014, 9:30 A.M.

SINCE YESTERDAY WAS SUCH A day of involved discipleship, I wanted to come back to the idea I have been exploring: how practicing discipleship now is good preparation for dying and death later. The practices and skills we engage in today as Christian disciples will become the habits of the heart that ease our transition from this life to the next and prepare us for life after death. In other words, we are practicing for heaven.

What are we practicing, exactly? What aspects of life in the here and now are going to carry forward into the next life? What are we going to be doing then that we can equip for now? I can think of at least three activities of thrilling activity in heaven: communing, worshipping, and reigning with Christ.

Communing. Finally, the veil will be lifted, and we will see Jesus, hear his voice, abide in his presence, and otherwise enjoy life with him. We will be back to the garden, where Adam and Eve roamed and where they bumped into God around every corner. Now we see through a glass darkly, but then we shall see him face to face. I can't wait. In the meantime, by the power of Christ's Spirit, we can actually learn to recognize the voice of Jesus and abide in his presence. Because Jesus's atoning death removed the barrier between God and us, we can commune with God at his table right now. The sacrament of the Lord's Supper, as an example, is one practice that prepares us for our eternity at the heavenly banquet (Luke 22:28ff).

Worshipping. Christians have told me they are worried that eternity in heaven will be boring. Citing harps and angels and insipid hymns, some folks think that joining a worshipping choir before God's throne will be something less than thrilling. I think this is more of a commentary on the worship in their home church; but if worship is boring now, they are going to have a startling awakening in the next life. The book of Revelation is full of heavenly worship scenes, with throngs united in praise, giving glory to our Creator and the Lamb on the Throne. If we are going to feel at home in that crowd, now is the time to start feeling at home with God's people, singing and praising the Lord and uniting in one purpose to give glory to Jesus Christ. This future suggests preparation in the present. We're going to be focused on God and singing his praises in heaven. Will we have the vocabulary, the voice, and the vitality for that? It's time to start practicing!

Reigning. This part of our job description in the presence of God kicks in after the mass resurrection of God's people, at the joining of the new heavens and the new earth, described so beautifully in the last few chapters of Revelation. Eternal life entails reigning with God over all his creation (Rev. 5:10, 22:5). We will be managing everything under God's authority, just as we were commissioned to do in the Garden of Eden (Gen. 1–2). This will be engaging, fulfilling, joyful work. It will require us to be very acquainted with God's economy, and our learning curve starts now as we discern how to participate in the kingdom of God in this life. This is the grand connection between this life and the next. We are practicing stewardship now—at home, at church, in the community—so that acting in partnership with God in heaven will be second nature to us. If we are faithful in the relatively little things God gives us to tend now, Jesus says we will be entrusted with much more responsibility later.

Practicing for heaven gives meaning and purpose to life, even as we approach death. Our present experience will be overshadowed by the Almighty in the world to come. If we are faithful in our practice today as citizens of the heavenly kingdom—in sickness and in health, in joy and in sorrow—our capacity to cooperate with God will be enhanced, and heaven will be a wonderful place for us. I believe this! That vision is what makes me willing and able to endure life, illness, and death. Even the deepest challenge provides an opportunity to practice for communing, worshipping, and reigning in the next life.

86 ✎

Surgery Scheduled for March 3

THURSDAY, JANUARY 23, 2014, 5 P.M.

IT'S OFFICIAL: I AM SCHEDULED for surgery on Monday, March 3. I'm thrilled about this news, most especially because I will be feeling fine the Friday night before, when Andy and I have a date to hear cellist Yo-Yo Ma and the San Francisco Symphony. After holding these tickets for a year and wondering if I will be able to go, it feels like a personal present from God.

87 &

Waiting to Die, or Living to Death?

FRIDAY, JANUARY 24, 2014

THREE YEARS AGO, ON THE occasion of her eightieth birthday, my mother stated that she was the longest living member of her family. Her vision of her life had not extended past that point, as every single one of her forebears had died early and suddenly or, in one case, at age seventy-two after a long illness. Since she does not know what to do with life after eighty and has no inclination to reinvent herself, it appears she is simply marking time and waiting to die. She is in perfect health, and I confess to thinking that this is going to be painful for other people to watch, because she is squandering a terrific opportunity for a meaningful season of life.

I came into church one Sunday alongside a dear lady who, at age one hundred, was walking from her residence down the street. To my cheerful greeting and inquiry as to her well-being, she replied, "I'm fine, but I don't know why I am still around." At that moment my job was to minister in Christ's name to a visionless person. It appeared that she—and perhaps even those who are content, fulfilled, or discouraged—needed a guide through life unto death, focusing not so much on the issue of dying as on the issue of living.

Regardless of our age or health status, what we do with the time we have left on this earth is the primary arena of our discipleship. We live in a now-but-not-yet situation: we know as Jesus followers that we possess eternal life, but we are not quite there yet. As long as we possess a perishable body, we cannot function fully within the realm of heaven. Or can we?

The core of our faith resides in the world of the eternal, even as we maintain residency in this tent (Paul's term, 2 Cor. 5:1–4). Are we not called to run this race with a vision of the inheritance awaiting us, as the writer of Hebrews so persuasively exhorted us (Heb. 12)? Did not Jesus persevere through his trial and crucifixion with a vision of joy set before him? What got Jesus over the hurdle of a horrible death was a vision of reigning with his heavenly Father. That vision enabled him to endure great pain and suffering and to fully live each moment until there were no moments left.

My thoughts have drifted in the direction of planning for the rest of my life. Since I am in the dark about my prognosis, I could have a few months or a couple of years left, or I could live to be in my nineties. Would I make different choices now if I knew I had only a few years to live? Would my priorities shift if I were assured that I had thirty years instead? The question has been teasing me.

It seems wise to make certain preparations for death and then to live each day as if on a thirty-year investment. Concretely, this means I am giving some thought to final arrangements—gathering ideas for a memorial service and gearing up to write an obituary (having ranted to my husband about the clichés and overused phrases I read in obits every day). Now would be the time to fill out a Five Wishes document, which spells out to family members and medical providers my preferences for end-of-life care, and an advance directive related to specific medical intervention under certain circumstances. This is the least I can do for my loved ones later.

But that's enough on end-of-life preparations.

How do I want to *live* in the meantime? What does it look like to live on a thirty-year investment? I am a planner by temperament and work style. At least five major projects lie envisioned, outlined, or mapped but incomplete on my desk. I operate in a swirl of unfinished business, like Pigpen in *Peanuts* walking around in a cyclone of dust. What is emerging for me is a desire to order my life in such a way as to get some of these projects done. I've certainly got thirty years of possibilities ahead of me; I want to live those experiences, projects, and explorations to the full. And I'd like to finish them if God would allow me time to do so. On the other hand, I wouldn't mind dying with an active Things To Do list on my desk.

This approach is not running away from reality; quite the contrary, I think, it is running toward life and embracing it fully. I most certainly want to live—not as an escape from dying but as preparation for it. Perhaps you have faced this more squarely and intimately than I am yet able to experience, but living fully until death seems to be the way to die. I can think of no better illustration of this than Roberto Benigni's character in the film *Life Is Beautiful*.

Guido, his wife, and their son, Joshua, are Jewish citizens sent to a German concentration camp in 1939. For the sake of his son, Guido, a clown by nature and wise in character, interprets what is happening as a game. Joshua has the opportunity to play for points, and if he wins he gets a military tank. By setting up the rules of the game and reinterpreting events as they occur, Guido shields his son from the horrors of what is happening and manages to help his son survive the ordeal. Guido, however, makes a critical mistake and is found out. Despite the approaching American liberation of the camp, Guido is led to his execution, but not before glimpsing his son one last time and keeping up the role of game player for him, right up until the end.

My intent is to live, fully and joyfully. Yes, I am going to die. Okay, so are you. When? Don't know, and I don't need to know. What I need to know I have in my possession already: a vision of life that is infused with joy, filled with the Spirit, empowered by God's grace, baited by good life-questions, and met with insatiable curiosity. I am going to keep living this life until God says, "Stop." If I ever ask you, "Why am I still around?" I expect you will have an answer, and it won't be some insipid platitude, because, starting now, you too are working on the answer to that question. Do not wait to die, but live to death, embracing fully both living and dying as stepping-stones to eternal life.

88 ✄

The Acceptance of Tragedy

SATURDAY, JANUARY 25, 2014

OUR NEWSPAPER HAS BEEN COVERING a tragic situation that warrants further reflection, in light of my comments on dying and death. A fourteen-year-old girl died from sudden complications after tonsil surgery. The state of California says she died—and I agree—because, in the course of this medical emergency, her brain ceased all functioning. All neurological activity in all areas of the brain ceased completely. However, as of today, she is still on a ventilator, which keeps her breathing and her heart beating. Her parents, holding religious beliefs only vaguely described to the media, do not believe she is dead as long as she has a heartbeat. The attorney representing the family is filing suit to secure for parents, rather than hospital or state, the legal right to determine when death has occurred in their minor children.

The case pushes the envelope of bioethics and is fueled by unspeakable parental grief and inability to accept a devastating tragedy. I have only the most profound compassion for the family and cannot imagine the anguish this situation causes them. However, I wonder what kind of counsel they are receiving about life and death. The fundamental, undergirding problem here is the denial of the reality of death and a failure to accept tragedy. This case epitomizes the bargaining stage of grief. It is cloaked in religious freedom issues, based on a belief that life ends not when the brain ceases to function but when the heart stops. The heroic measures are terribly misguided.

Our culture is finding it more difficult to accept tragedy as a part of life. People die. Many die suddenly because of accident or error. They die young. They die at the hand of another. A nation that has buried thousands of victims of mass tragedies—9/11, Oklahoma City, Sandy Hook—finds it difficult in *individual* cases to accept a definition of death because it can be trumped by the use of life-support machines.

Let's be clear: miracles happen. God is able to raise the dead. Keeping a teenager on a ventilator is not required for God to do what God is capable of doing. But God has not resuscitated the patient, so when is it time to give up and accept the tragedy? Do parents think they are acting in the best interest of their child? Or are they begrudging her transition from this life to the next? Their daughter is dead, and her soul has left her body to be with the Lord. Meanwhile, her parents, as people of faith, are unhappy about *that*? It is so unspeakably sad that these bereaved parents cannot acknowledge a passage that sets their daughter free from the trials and sickness of this life—and liberates them to remember her and move on.

Deep pain accompanies our conclusion that a tragedy has unfolded, a life has been lost, and there is nothing more that can be done about it. But it is part of the discipleship process to accept what will not change and to surrender to the gracious heart of God. Then we can truly grieve, joyfully remember, and purposefully live into the future and all the days God has numbered for us to live.

89 ✑

Fitness Goals for February

MONDAY, JANUARY 27, 2014

THIS WEEKEND ANDY AND I tested our hiking muscles on a couple of outings. Oh, gee, am I out of shape! It felt good to get a cardio workout—the old ticker and lungs doing just fine—but, surprisingly, my general muscle tone is shot. I haven't begun to test core strength, but I suspect it and the arms need a good workout too.

While I'm off treatment the next month, I hope to regain some muscle tone in time for surgery, so I am devising a sensible plan for gradual rebuilding. I've been a goal setter for decades, since my first pregnancy, when my objective was to go the full distance in labor completely naturally and without pain medications. I prepared for delivery like an athlete and walked three miles the day Katy was born.

In the Before Cancer (BC) days, I hiked a minimum of forty-five minutes every day on hills in our Open Space, plus two gym workouts per week for strength and muscle toning. I haven't been able to do this since returning from Africa last August, the longest exercise hiatus in about ten years. So I have devised a plan for incremental progress, with hiking-pace goals and exercise repetitions mapped out.

The fatigue I feel while walking is unique; I tell Andy I feel it at the cellular level. Winded, yes—which simply demonstrates some cardio build up is necessary—but I am also anemic and white-cell compromised. Care and persistence are called for, and getting out in this beautiful spring weather benefits soul and body.

90 ✍

The Lost Keys

SOMEWHERE LAST FALL I LOST my car keys and accompanying house key. It happened while I was still in the hubbub of unpacking from our Africa vacation, switching purses, re-organizing for normal life, and finding out about my cancer.

For a long time, I said, "They must be around here someplace. They will turn up." But coping with radiation and chemo was consuming. Cancer patients talk about "chemo brain," a fuzzy-headed inability to keep thoughts flowing and retain memory. I don't think I ever had that condition, although not being able to find my keys gave evidence to the contrary. After searching all my pockets, retracing steps, and otherwise turning the house upside down looking for them, I gave up on the keys by Christmas.

Life went on. Last Friday night my husband and I decided it was time to try a couple of modest hikes to assess my strength and stamina. The trails were anticipated to be dry and dusty—really, summer conditions around here—so I decided to get out my lightweight hiking pants.

You guessed it. As I unfurled the pants, out dropped my car keys. Their familiar little clatter was music to my ears. I hooted and screamed in delight, relieved that they had been in a "safe" place all this time.

I identify with the woman in Jesus's parable about the lost coin (Luke 15:8–10). She focused on her search, scrutinized and swept every corner, searching high and low for something of value to her. And when she found it, she called together her friends and neighbors to celebrate. Jesus used this ordinary life occurrence to illustrate the joy in heaven when one sinner repents. To God we are like the lost coin.

God searches for us when we get lost spiritually, and all of heaven rejoices when we turn around to be found by him. Our lostness is of deep concern to God. He has gone to great lengths to find us and bring us back where we belong. His search is motivated by love and owner-ship, in the sense that we, along with all of God's creation, are his. We belong to God. We are cherished by God and missed when we assert our independence and walk out of fellowship with him. God embraces and forgives us as we turn around, leave our errant path, and face the Savior. This turning around goes by the word *repentance*.

The first time I truly repented, I was seventeen and gripped by the gospel of Jesus Christ. I have repented many times since, as God has shown me those areas where I have served myself instead of him, where I have embraced a habit more tightly than him, where I have asserted my way contrary to his. The great turnaround underway in this season of my life is from busy blindness to contemplative reflection, from feeling driven to being called. There's a lot of rejoicing in heaven yet to come, as these transformations are built into my life.

How about you? Are you suffering from spiritual "chemo brain," forgetting where you have put your faith? Are you lost in any area of your life, wandering off the path, distracted into disobedience? Are you asserting independence or self-reliance, rebuffing God's grace and help? You realize—don't you?—that unrepentance is postponing a great party in heaven, not to mention the redemption of that part of your life.

I'm really glad I found my keys. I'm even more glad that God found me and has been working his transformation in me all these years. But my joy is miniscule compared to the ecstatic celebration God is hosting as one of his own repents and returns to the party.

91 ⬿

People Need Some Good News

Thursday, January 30, 2014

YESTERDAY I GOT TO MEET with my "Peet's ladies," fellow gym enthu-
siasts who gather daily for coffee at Peet's after their workouts. It was
a joyful reunion. We sat down for a cup and caught up with each other.
My prayer list for each one was updated, and they were encouraged to see
me with their own eyes and to know that I was doing well.

Since November, I have had a steady parade of home visits from
friends, almost all of whom know the Lord and bring the Spirit's comfort
and companionship to me. But I have missed the Peet's ladies—the one
group in my life that does not know Christ—and their nonstop chatter
about anything and everything. Turns out, they missed me too.

The talk quickly turned to how well I am doing, and it is as natural
as sharing a yummy recipe to tell them that God is at work to bring me
healing. I am utterly convinced that the Lord is going to complete the
work that has been started by the doctors' administrations of chemo and
radiation. I believe God has shown mercy through the aggressive treatment assault upon my body, its effectiveness at shrinking the tumor, the
lack of serious nausea or utter misery, the manageable and short-duration
discomfort associated with radiation, and my short recovery time between treatments. Some may call this incredibly good luck, but given the
norm for cases like mine, I sense that God has intervened on my behalf

in a remarkable way. So I am verbalizing it to anyone celebrating with me the progress toward complete healing.

As I move from one social circle to another, I am giving witness not only of a sterling medical team, but also of God's unique and powerful activity. It is surprisingly easy to share about God in this context because he is so close and real and the results so tangible. Others to whom I speak are encouraged, as they see a living, breathing example of trusting Jesus and the power of prayer. To God be the glory!

When Jesus commissioned us to be his witnesses and to make disciples (Matt. 28:19f), he opened the door for us to share what God is doing in our lives. The first disciples—former fishermen and tax collectors—boldly shared testimony to Jesus Christ in the power of the Spirit. What would have been impossible three years prior had become an everyday activity: to lift up the name of Jesus and share an enthusiastic story of what he had done.

So what holds us back from bringing up the Lord's goodness in a conversation with those unacquainted with God's mercy? I can think of a few possibilities.

We are out of touch with God's activity in our lives and on our behalf. This is a surprisingly powerful deterrent to Christian witnessing: we do not pause to reflect on what God is doing; consequently we do not give thanks nor give God glory. We are so preoccupied with finding our own solutions to God-sized problems that we miss the clues that point to our Savior. This is why it is important that we rehearse frequently the story of our conversion, or our discovery of Christ's presence in our lives, or a turning point of repentance. Never forget what the Lord has done for you and what good news it really is. "Bless the LORD, O my soul, and do not forget all his benefits!" (Ps. 103:2).

We have put our faith in a private compartment that we feel shouldn't be opened in public. Part of this dynamic is the belief that spiritual things are only internal, and therefore very personal. We believe their impact is not visible nor of interest to the casual observer. But, wow, doesn't the Christian faith change a person from the inside out? Is our faith irrelevant to everyday living? Is our faith powerless to express itself in a visible, active way? If faith is woven into our everyday life, it is going to show. You might as well let people know why you have an uncommon joy in the face of adversity, or why you have been able to move on after a disaster, or who was behind your healing. People want to know, and I am impressed with my friends for showing me respect and sharing my joy at what God is doing.

We overthink how people might react when we mention Jesus. This is the fear category. We are afraid, for instance, that people might think us kooky if we give credit to Jesus for what they think is accomplished only by medical science. But our testimony simply offers an alternative, very viable interpretation of what is happening, something our unbelieving friends may not have considered before. Even if I were to die today, my Peet's ladies would know God gave me joy and serenity in this cancer experience. They would know I considered God a partner in the medical practice of my doctors. They would know I had lived life confidently because God was trustworthy. I am not afraid of what they might think, because what God is doing is real, and they can see it. When we share our experience transparently and authentically, others have an opportunity to see what God is like in real life.

92 🌿

A Turning Point in Prayer

MONDAY, FEBRUARY 3, 2014

IN THE "FOR WHAT IT'S WORTH" department, I had an interesting experience while in prayer this morning. I'm not sure what to make of it. I was going through my usual list of prayer requests for family, friends, and world concerns and was about to close with my request for healing of this cancer. But the Lord interrupted me before I could ask. It was a "verbal sense"—not an audible voice, but a strong intruding thought, clearly distinguishable from my thoughts at that moment. The Lord said, "Ah, Mary, you don't need to pray about that anymore. It's done."

93 🍃

Fading Glory

B Y ALL ACCOUNTS, MY RECOVERY from the negative effects of chemo round 3 has been unusually quick and thorough, much more so than my recovery from round two. I am hiking at least two miles a day now to build up my strength and to regain cardiopulmonary endurance for surgery on March 3. God has been very good to suppress the queasiness or sleepiness I had in previous rounds, and it is nice to say life is getting back to normal. The drugs continue to create an extremely inhospitable environment for the Beast in my body, if there is any life in it yet, which I doubt.

One drug in my infusion protocol is a mixed bag, so to speak. It is a steroid designed to amplify the effectiveness of the antinausea drugs. Its side effects include a frustrating twenty-pound weight gain and serendipitous joint pain relief. Two weeks out from the last infusion, I am feeling my normal joint discomforts, a signal that the steroid is finally wearing off. I must pay attention once again to body mechanics and stretching exercises, along with my walking/hiking routine, to maintain physical comfort, especially in that pesky right shoulder. Despite my love-hate relationship with the drug, I'm sorry to see this one positive side effect fade.

The people of God can experience a similar spiritual "wearing off" effect, simply because of the limitations of our human existence. We humans are touched with God's healing presence and power, but the effects of these close encounters often fade. Our eyes grow dim to the glory of God, we slip back into bad habits, we come down off the mountaintop, only to stumble over something in the valley. It is safe to say that just about every stellar Bible character experienced the comedown in one way or another. It is as if all of us are subject to a spiritual force of gravity that pulls us earthward, away from the freeing effects of God's love and power.

Moses had his moments of spiritual ecstasy—face-to-face encounters with the living God in the tabernacle. He would go in to meet God on a regular basis and come out with such an extraordinary glow on his face that he wore a veil to keep from blinding the Israelites (Ex. 34:33f). What the people didn't know was that the veil also hid the fading of that glorious light. Moses was enamored with the status symbol that accompanied his special access to the Almighty. According to Paul in 2 Corinthians 3:7–18, Moses kept the veil on long after the glory had faded, to create the lasting impression that elevated his reputation among the people. All he was hiding was his humanity, which limits one's capacity to hold on to the blessings of God. It's as if we leak; there are holes in us, making it impossible to stay filled with the glory of God.

Paul's only answer to this problem of spiritual leakage is to rely upon the daily infilling of the Holy Spirit. It's like managing a slow oil leak in an old car; sometimes it's more cost effective to replace a quart of oil than it is to do the big expensive repair job. While we live on this earth, our spiritual life will have holes in it. But the Lord's mercies (and power) are new every morning, calling us to be filled once again (Lam. 3:22f). What would otherwise fade in us—the faith, hope, and love of our Savior and the glory of Almighty God—is renewed every day by the power of the Holy Spirit.

Relying on God's Spirit keeps us on the path, and his Word is a light unto our feet (Ps. 119:105). Abandoning either Word or Spirit places us in a perilous position, though it might take a long time to see the full effect of faded glory. Maintaining spiritual discipline, including study of God's Word, is important for retaining our strength and spiritual health in the days to come. To those who strive to foster these spiritual habits, I offer encouragement and prayers for your continued faithfulness to Jesus Christ and the fullness of his Spirit. For those who do not, the discipline may be painful in the short term, but later will yield "the peaceful fruit of righteousness" (Heb. 12:11).

I also want to put aside any desire to wear a veil of false glory and instead allow the vulnerabilities of cancer—and mortal humanity—to show. There is no shame in admitting that cancer can suck the life out of me and turn my facial tone to gray some days. But daily visits with my heavenly Father and great Physician keep me in a good, honest, and redeemed place, where I can savor the life of this day and trust him for the future.

94 🍂

Mother's Offer

MY EIGHTY-THREE-YEAR-OLD MOTHER CALLED YESTERDAY with an offer to travel from Washington to stay with us in California for a few days. She sounded tentative, and I must admit, I was surprised that she would even entertain the idea. Probing gently, I discerned that her friends had recommended the trip as a way to comfort her worry.

"Wow, Mom, that would be so nice of you to come. Do you feel you are up to a trip?"

"I think you could use some help."

"I would love it if you wanted to come help, Mom. I'm pretty much stuck in my recliner these days."

"I'm slowing down, myself . . ."

"Mom, you know that if you came, I wouldn't be able to entertain you, right? That you would be making yourself available to help me rather than the other way around? Are you up to it?"

Quiet.

"How would you like to travel?" A decades-long fear of flying eliminated that mode of transportation, but Mom had taken a driving trip with a friend last summer and used to love to take the train.

"Would you enjoy the Starlight Super? Andy could pick you up at the train station in Martinez."

"Well, I wouldn't want to go alone."

"I bet you could arrange for [my brother] Mike to accompany you, or maybe one of your girlfriends would enjoy a train trip down the coast."

Her hesitancy was audible.

"Mom, why don't we both sleep on this idea and talk again tomorrow. Think about what scenario would work for you. The guest room here is ready, and we could welcome you at the drop of a hat. Just say when and how."

I felt a great tenderness toward this strong but fearful lady. I haven't heard from her today, and it doesn't seem possible that she could work out in her worried mind how to make the eight-hundred-mile trip. But she gave it a valiant try.

95 ✑

Under the Weather

THURSDAY, FEBRUARY 6, 2014

AS THE WEATHER TURNS GRAY and rainy, I have been under the weather myself: body achy, throat scratchy, and voice dropping an octave. Although I slept well, I woke up this morning without a voice. Time to hunker down and shake off this bug.

But it isn't all that clear cut. Sometimes I feel like a walking chemistry experiment. So many things going on in my body could cause various symptoms. Some possible causes occur to me:

- The steroids are wearing off, which probably contributes to the joint aches.
- I've been exercising pretty hard. I may have overdone it a bit, overtaxing my body's self-healing abilities.
- I went to church on Sunday and got a lot of hugs. People self-select and stay clear if they know they are sick, but one can be contagious before one feels symptoms. Perhaps I picked something up.
- A little tightness and congestion in the chest suggests possible inflammation at the radiation site. I hope it runs its course without any future complications.

Otherwise, I am very encouraged. My mind is stimulated by some interesting church-related work this week, I've completed some sewing (including getting to the bottom of the mending pile), and I have books to read and people to see. I certainly am not feeling lonely or bored, and Andy is finding interesting, local adventures each weekend to keep me in touch with the wider world. What a blessing he is to me.

96 ✑

Hanging On to Hope

MONDAY, FEBRUARY 10, 2014

MY BUG EVOLVED FROM A scratchy throat to laryngitis, a cough, and a low-grade fever. It was probably something I picked up at church last weekend, so I stayed home this weekend to avoid germs. It's hard to believe that seven days ago I was hiking over two miles per day and feeling wonderful and optimistic. Since Wednesday, my dominant feelings have been lethargy, discomfort, and concern as my symptoms accumulated. Lung cancer makes one a bit skittish about what would otherwise be normal winter blahs.

It has been just three months since my diagnosis, and since then I have undergone three rounds of chemotherapy and 45-Gray (4500 rads) of radiation. In those months of active treatment, God met me at a very tender place and carried me through the discomforts of a rigorous routine. It was as if I were resting in our backyard hammock once again. Just last week I had a very palpable sense that God was healing me, and I rejoiced.

But the proactive fight has morphed into dull waiting. The novelty and initial challenge of this experience has passed. I am now in the midst of five weeks without doctors' appointments, infusions, and tests. The waiting routine consists of the slow, steady climb toward strength and fitness in preparation for surgery—nothing really exciting about that, just uphill, ordinary life.

And then I started to cough again, which summoned scary memories of last fall. For three days I gutted it out, somewhat discouraged and tired, a bit beat up spiritually. Late Friday afternoon my pastor was visiting and praying for me when the Lord seemed to nudge me. His word was, "The fact that you feel sick again doesn't change what I am accomplishing in you. Don't let this momentary setback rob you of the hope I have given you. Keep your eyes on the goal, and let my joy be your strength!"

This feverish stupor has led me to reflect on how my experience parallels that of the people of God in New Testament history: early exuberance, fruitful ministry, doldrums and difficulties, followed by strengthened hope.

The early chapters of Acts describe how those who had witnessed Jesus's resurrection—or heard about it directly from his disciples—were high on the gospel. God used Spirit-empowered but otherwise ordinary men and women to tell the story, heal, forgive, and evangelize. Nothing could stop them, and miracles were many. They were energized not only by past events, such as Pentecost, but by a future hope: the imminent return of their beloved friend and Savior, Jesus. They embraced the challenge of the Great Commission, and their new life in Christ motivated them to remain faithful to the task.

As decades passed, they held on to that hope, even though Christ did not return in their lifetimes. Then the Roman persecution started, endangering a new generation of believers and tempting them to forget the hope that rested within them. Many died with "Maranatha—Come, Lord!" on their lips and the hope of the resurrection in their hearts. Some died as martyrs. But none saw Jesus return in glory. What carried them was faith, "the assurance of things hoped for, the conviction of things not seen" (Heb. 11:1).

You may have started out, as I did, feeling that you could do all things through Christ who strengthened you, only to have the glow wear off after a few months or years. My sense is that God gently withdraws some of the exciting aspects of Christian experience over time in order to increase our trust in the ordinary, steadfast love of God. This is part of the process of Christian maturing that builds our faith and enables us to endure the ups and downs of life, the boredom of waiting periods, and the weight of responsibility within the kingdom. Time in "the waiting room" comes with the territory, as do earthly afflictions like cancer that remind us to hang on to the hope that does not disappoint. I am trying to keep this in mind when the day's circumstances pull me under a cloud. Jesus is sustaining me and giving meaning to my existence. With this God-view, all of life looks a lot different.

97

Fever Develops

MONDAY, FEBRUARY 10, 2014

SPENT THE DAY IN BED yesterday with a fever and a chest cough with lots of congestion. My voice comes and goes. I am waiting for the oncologist's office to open this morning and will call for advice. Can't let this develop into full-blown anything, since surgery is three weeks away.

Bed Rest and Amoxicillin

TUESDAY, FEBRUARY 11, 2014

WAS SEEN YESTERDAY BY THE nurse practitioner, who dispensed appropriate sympathy and skill. She took one look at my throat and said she suspected strep throat—an opportunistic infection under these conditions—and decided to start me on amoxicillin right away. The fever came down overnight, and I am hoping to be fever-free day today. Meanwhile, I'm staying close to bed and doing all the prudent things— drinking lots of fluids, taking acetaminophen—to whip this bug. Such bad timing, right before surgery!

Fever Gone, but Not the Blahs

THURSDAY, FEBRUARY 13, 2014

THE FEVER IS GONE, THANK the Lord. So today I will take a flat walk around the neighborhood and begin the slow climb to fitness once again. I am feeling depressed about my pudgy body, and I sigh in anticipation of the work it is going to take to get back into shape. After so many wonderful victories the last three months, this feels like an ignominious defeat. I don't think this is coming from vanity as much as a desire to feel well. First things first—getting over this bug—then perhaps another day I can tackle the larger challenge of weight loss and overall fitness. A person can fight only so many battles at the same time.

Not Even Blahs Now...

SUNDAY, FEBRUARY 16, 2014

STILL TAKING MY ANTIBIOTIC, BUT I am definitely on the mend, without complications. Yesterday, slowly but surely, I conquered Flat Top and today followed up with a fast flat mile. Otherwise I play this very conservatively and occupy myself with quiet pursuits, such as completing the Sunday *New York Times* crossword puzzle in ninety minutes this morning. I think that's my record. All is well, and God is holding me up.

98 ✑

Another "Come to Jesus" Moment

Life in slow motion is giving me the opportunity to revisit issues, temptations, and directions of my past life as a pastor. Today the theme is fatigue, which I have felt persistently now for weeks. Weeks ago my doctors prepared me for the possibility that the negative effects of chemo and radiation could sneak up on me well after the treatment period was over. Ever the optimist, I imagined this chemo hiatus would allow almost six weeks of steady strengthening. Instead it has turned out to be a disappointing holding pattern. Last week I had a short-term setback in the form of "the crud" morphing into strep throat. All this is to say I'm tired, really tired.

I've been exhausted in previous seasons of life: the year our new church building was under construction and it felt like we planned everything twice (Plan A and Plan B); or the year nine people in my congregation died between Thanksgiving and Christmas; or the seventy-hour work weeks and all-nighters at peak times. Yes, the life of a pastor is demanding and often exhausting.

But nothing like the exhaustion felt at the cellular level that I am experiencing now. I can report from personal experience that the full-on assault designed to vanquish the Beast has also done a number on *me*. I should be glad for this, because it is proof that the weapons of medical science are on a seek-and-destroy mission throughout my body. Despite the fatigue, I have a strong sense that the Beast has been slain already. We'll get confirmation of that when I have lung surgery on March 3. But while I wait for that good word, I am required to draw strength not from my own powers but from another source.

God seems to be offering a "Come to Jesus" moment. While I use this phrase humorously, it is literally true. Whenever I feel the weight of tiredness, it is as if the Lord is speaking directly to me the words of Jesus in Matthew's gospel: "Come to me, all you that are weary and are carrying heavy burdens, and I will give you rest" (Matt. 11:28).

Coming to Jesus at that very moment of weariness is both a skill and a privilege of the Christian life. It is natural, for someone as proud and strong as I have been, to want to hide from Jesus in moments of weakness or fatigue. Humans are tempted put on masks to cover their inadequacies with hope of making themselves presentable to God.

But there is no use hiding our true condition from the one who sees us as we really are. Jesus invites us to come to him right now. We don't have to wait until we feel better, until matters are more under control, or until we feel we've done our part (whatever that could possibly be) to gain God's favor. When Jesus said "Come to me and I will give you rest," he was saying the only way we can be strengthened through our entire being is by his gracious, gentle presence tenderly expressing God's love for us.

Getting to that place of quietness and trust comes with practice. I was not so good at releasing my fatigue into Jesus's care in my early years as a pastor. While I am not completely there yet, I know that I am hearing Jesus's voice more clearly and responding more readily in the "Come to Jesus" moments.

99 ✐

Come to the Waters

Saturday, February 22, 2014

As I continue to struggle with fatigue, I recall my early days of motherhood, before the babies were sleeping through the night. How many months can a person go without uninterrupted sleep? With our first daughter, God had mercy on us in six weeks, after which we could get seven or eight hours straight. But our second daughter was still waking up in the middle of the night at five months. I remember being so completely exhausted in September 1983 that I canceled my involvement in every single activity. I was grouchy and desperate for relief. "This, too, passed," but not before I had seen the ugly side of my spirituality—anger at God, losing my grip on faith—and realized what a fair-weather friend I was to God.

That's when I simply had to put into action God's invitation to "Come, all you who are thirsty, come to the waters" (Isa. 55:1). My very ordered 5:30 a.m.-like-clockwork quiet time went by the wayside and was replaced by many short stops during the day to draw water from the Lord's well. Even as I drink tap water to keep the body in motion, I drink of the living water to keep the soul alive and well. My sips during the day included recalling from memory Scriptures of encouragement and comfort, reading a psalm or two, quieting my soul for centering prayer, or listening to music "that soothes the savage breast."

Thirty years later, what was then a desperate plan to stay in touch with

God has become a sweet and refreshing method of regaining strength in the middle of a different kind of exhaustion—cancer fatigue. What I learned then I cherish now: God loves to provide living water from his inexhaustible source so I can stay spiritually hydrated. This is what Jesus meant, I think, when he said to the Samaritan woman at the well:

> Everyone who drinks of this [well] water will be thirsty again, but those who drink of the water that I will give them will never be thirsty. The water that I will give will become in them a spring of water gushing up to eternal life. (John 4:13f)

Lately I have received deep drafts of living water from friends who come to visit or send cards of encouragement. They have no idea how far these simple gestures go to quench spiritual thirst and empower me to rest.

So let's meet at the well, shall we? Whatever the source of your fatigue, come to the water that gushes up to eternal life!

100 𝒶

Come in Weakness

In decades past, tiredness of the usual kind was remedied by sleep, because the cause was hard work, long days, or stress. Anyone denied sleep because of work's demands experiences a sleep deficit. The only way to pay it back is to sleep.

The other kind of fatigue—the kind I am experiencing now—is remedied by healing. My body, exerting hidden energy, is fighting an infection and undergoing chemotherapy and/or radiation. I hope the stress on my immune system will abate as the underlying condition is healed. This healing certainly requires medicine. But it also takes time. For me, the process involves extra sleep (sleeping in until 7:30 or 8:00 most days, as well as taking afternoon naps).

Either way, in fatigue we experience weakness and vulnerability. But in the past I have invested a lot in *not* being weak or vulnerable. I am a firstborn overachiever, a wife and mother in demand for so many ordinary things, and a woman in leadership in a male-dominated field. People see me as the strong one in challenging situations. I do not give up ground easily.

The question is, how are we to *be* when exhaustion, sickness, or some other defeat renders us too tired to *do*? Since weakness (or its sister, powerlessness) is so debilitating, we may not be able to fix it, but the Bible offers insight for getting through it.

The apostle Paul had a nagging problem he called his "thorn in the flesh" (2 Cor. 12). We don't know what it was, but it weakened him. Paul believed that God had allowed it so that he would not get puffed up by the special spiritual visions and visitations he had experienced. He repeatedly asked God to remove this thorn, but finally the resolution came in a word: "My grace is sufficient for you, for power is made perfect in weakness." With that, Paul resolved to "boast all the more gladly of my weaknesses, so that the power of Christ may dwell in me" (2 Cor. 12:9).

Eugene Peterson renders this verse, "My grace is enough; it's all you need. My strength comes into its own in your weakness" (MSG). Paul was discovering that the remedy for his weakness was God's strength. He was finally able to accept that gift and not worry about being weak in the flesh.

Having experienced a concentrated four months of weakness, I think I am getting this. When we finally give in and say, "Okay, Lord, I am confronted with my limitations and realize how totally dependent I am upon you," we give God soul-room to work his mighty power in our spirit. The very thing we have proudly identified as strength has, in reality, allowed us to resist the gentle infusion of God's patience and power. It is so much better to admit our true condition, receive inner strength from the Great Physician, and thank God for being our one and only Savior.

It is amazing to me how the very act of standing down and resting creates the sort of spiritual vacuum that Jesus then fills with himself. The hammock moment last fall, when I felt carried by God, was when I discovered this place of deep rest. It became possible for me to move through this illness as Jesus took over. In personal surrender I could align with God's purposes rather than play field marshal and order God to stand in formation according to my "strong" plan. My limitations have become one arena for God's unlimited power to shine through, so that someday it may be said of me, "It was not Mary you saw, but Christ in her" (from Gal. 2:20).

101 ✒

All Systems "Go" for Surgery

TUESDAY, FEBRUARY 25, 2014

ANDY AND I WENT TO see Dr. Chen for a pre-op checkup. Everything looks good going into surgery. My blood numbers are up (platelets and white count especially), and my lungs continue to sound very good. So we're a go for next Monday.

My continuing fatigue is to be expected and no cause for alarm. The cough that has become more pronounced the last few days is a side effect of the radiation, and it too is nothing to worry about. I get winded more easily for the same reason, but I am to do what I can to "keep filling my lungs with air." I realize that *singing* would be good exercise, along with my walks.

Dr. Chen said it is not unusual for short-term muscle recovery after exercise to take two to three times longer than normal. So I shall reduce my hiking schedule from daily to twice a week. Just keep filling my lungs. Right now our one flight of stairs at home winds me.

Surgery is scheduled for 8:30 a.m. on Monday, March 3, at John Muir Walnut Creek. The plan is to remove the entire upper left lobe of the lung, including the tumor that remains, plus the neighboring lymph nodes. The surgeon hopes this can be done through a two-inch incision in my side. I'll be in the intensive care unit overnight, then in a regular room for up to five days in the hospital. I am looking forward to having both daughters here from Seattle to be with Andy and me on surgery day. Once I get home I will have the help of my aunt, a retired nurse, who will keep an eye on my recovery for a few days. Then my friends will help out for another few weeks until I can lift things and drive again.

102 🍃

Check-in with the Surgeon

FRIDAY, FEBRUARY 28, 2014

MY SURGEON CALLED LATE YESTERDAY afternoon and answered a few more questions before Monday's procedure. She said it would be fairly short, about two hours, but with preambles, preps, and travel time, I will be in in the surgery department for four hours. After the nurses in Recovery give the green light, I will be wheeled to ICU overnight for observation. Then the project is learning how to breathe again minus a lung lobe. A nurse called to talk to me about pain management, reassuring me this is nothing like labor and delivery! All the insurance red tape has been cut, managed, anticipated, approved . . . This is beginning to feel like a big deal.

So what's a girl to do? Tonight Andy and I are venturing over to San Francisco to hear Yo-Yo Ma in concert with the San Francisco Symphony.

103 🌿

Offering a Song in Gratitude

SUNDAY, MARCH 2, 2013

THIS MORNING AT CHURCH, I took the opportunity to share how faithful God has been during the last few months. I have appreciated the expressions of his love through these people who have been wonderful to us. Not knowing if I will be able to sing again after tomorrow's lung-altering surgery, I sang "Give Me Jesus" as my offering of praise. All two octaves of Moses Hogan's arrangement came through beautifully. To God be the glory.

I'm ready to get the show on the road. God is close and comforting, and I am not fearful or anxious. Just ready!

104 🌿

Surgery Went Well

Monday, March 3, 2014, 2:31pm

Andy here . . . Just spoke with Mary's surgeon. Mary is out of surgery and in recovery. The surgeon feels great about how it went. Plan A was achieved since the tumor had not attached itself to the mediastinum. The Beast is removed for good!

Mary will be moved to ICU in a bit, as per plan. Katy, Judy, and I are feeling great about the news! Woohoo!

Smiling Mary

Monday, March 3, 2014, 5:46pm

Andy again . . . Saw Mary in ICU an hour ago, and she was resting, talking, laughing, coughing, wincing, and hitting the button for painkillers. On course.

105 ⌒

Cotton Mouth

MONDAY, MARCH 3, 2014

DAY 1 POST-OP: MORPHINE IS a very fine medicine and effective pain-killer. It doesn't reach everything, like the persistent back spasm gripping my left shoulder blade, but it manages every other pain I'm experiencing quite well, thank you.

Nevertheless, morphine has a few side effects, most notably dry mouth. When I woke from the anesthesia and my daughters Katy and Judy came to see me in ICU, my mouth was completely dry, to the point of sticking to itself. Talking through a wad of cotton was impossible, eliciting polite giggles from the girls, who were struggling to catch what I was saying.

"Bribe a nurse, and get me some ice chips, please." Apparently it was a little too soon after surgery for the medical staff to let me ingest liquids, but the situation was getting quite desperate. Katy and Judy were gone a few minutes and came back with a precious two teaspoons of ice chips, which they began to feed me one at a time. Relief! Happiness! Thankfulness! All is right with the world! Okay, I can do this.

Dry mouth is a little different from thirst, I think, but relief comes with the same remedy: water. What ran through my head was the psalmist's description of spiritual thirst:

O God, you are my God, I seek you,
>   my soul thirsts for you;
>   my flesh faints for you,
>   as in a dry and weary land where there is no water.
(Psalm 63:1)

In Israel (and California), where water is a very precious commodity, people understand the physical craving for liquid across their lips. But David the psalmist is identifying a spiritual thirst, which may have accompanied a period of trial or even the dark night of the soul, in which he craved contact with the living God. David's soul clings in desperation to the Lord, because if he lets go, he knows the surrounding desert will swallow him.

Many of us feel the world sucks us dry. We exert every ounce of energy to take care of our families, be earnest workers, pay the mortgage. We go through seasons that feel like all output with no input. We pour out our lives in these efforts but receive nothing back to refill the well. All we know is that we are barely surviving.

God says, "Come to the waters, and drink of me!" (Isa. 55:1). Do we realize how close to spiritual dehydration we are? Physically, a headache is the first sign that I haven't had enough water today. Spiritually, my clue is deadened senses to the presence and power of God. What sates this thirst? Quiet time in the presence of Jesus, meditating on his Word, receiving spiritual refreshment from his inexhaustible supply. In other words, coming to the fountain and drinking in the Spirit of God. We might adopt a healthier spiritual habit if, when we take a glass of water (literally), we give thanks for Jesus and his living water too. And ask, "Lord, what part of me is withering for lack of spiritual refreshment?" This is the sort of question Jesus delights to answer because he is ready to pour into us whatever will keep us going. So, cheers!

106 🍃

Pain Management—Part 1

Day 2 post-op: My comfort level rose overnight. I have been moved to a spacious private room with a view of Mt. Diablo. Pain is under control, and I even sang a bit to test the pipes. At the way-too-early hour of 6:30 this morning I was encouraged to sit up in a chair, and I feasted on a regular breakfast.

Pain management is a major focus of surgical care. A few days prior to my surgery, a nurse called to explain how pain is controlled. Her message was important for me to hear since I have a tendency to opt out of pain meds. She said, "Don't be a hero; take the meds!"

The night before my early-morning appearance at the hospital, the anesthesiologist specializing in nerve blocks called me to explain the purpose and method of his procedure. The idea was to deaden certain nerves to give local pain relief during and after surgery, reducing the need for morphine, which tends to suppress respiration. After I arrived at the hospital early yesterday morning, I demonstrated a rather dramatic intolerance to the nerve block (I fainted—oops), so it was Plan B (morphine) for me and another opportunity to trust God.

When you wake up after a major surgery like this and cough that first time, you know why your caregivers are concerned about pain control. I was hooked up to an IV dispensing 10 mg of slow-drip morphine per day, and the nurse handed me a Patient Controlled Analgesia (PCA) button to push whenever I needed an extra boost of pain relief. This arrangement has managed the situation quite nicely for the first twenty-four hours. When the nurses realized I wasn't using the PCA anymore, they switched over to a nonsteroid anti-inflammatory called Toradol, which should work great for another twenty-four hours.

107 🍃

Unbind Her and Let Her Go!

WEDNESDAY, MARCH 5, 2014

DAY THREE POST-OP: SINCE MONDAY evening following my surgery, I have been tethered to my bed. Eleven different ties held me down: automatic leg compressors wrapped around my calves, a surgical drain from my side, a catheter, a blood-pressure cuff, five leads adhered to my torso for the EKG and respiration counter, an IV in each hand, a peripherally inserted central catheter (PICC line), and an oxygen cannula stuck in my nose. These various input and output devices gave medical staff signals as to my well-being and access for further treatment. They kept various bodily functions in balance. I am grateful for each one. But I was also captive.

Tuesday morning my big field trip was the few steps to the bathroom. But this required unhooking, unplugging, and a nurse in attendance to keep remaining tubes and cables from getting tangled. My entourage and I were quite a sight.

The surgeon visited after lunch, took one look at me, and decided it was time to get me moving around. She ordered all the paraphernalia detached and removed, everything but one IV line. Wow! Freedom!

Actually, what came to mind was Lazarus, called out of the grave by his friend Jesus (John 11:41–44). Just after his invitation of "Lazarus, come out!" Jesus commanded, "Unbind him and let him go!" In those moments after rising from the grave, Lazarus was alive, healthy, and yet tightly bound by the grave cloths. To get on with the new life Jesus had just given back to him, someone had to untether him.

In day-to-day life, of course, many things tether us physically, emotionally, and spiritually: hunger or addiction; vengeance, grief, or greed; guilt or shame, for starters. A fixation on the past can tether us, and fear of the future can grip us even more. The fact is, our human condition without Jesus Christ is enslavement of one kind or another, until we are redeemed and transformed by our Savior. A personal examination, with the help of the Holy Spirit, can lead to awareness of the bindings gripping our soul. We are to "lay aside every weight and the sin that clings so closely, and . . . run with perseverance the race that is set before us" (Heb. 12:1). Only then do we have complete freedom, the freedom to live righteously in unhindered fellowship with God. The dangers of entanglement are everywhere, but Jesus's voice, if heeded, will lead us away from dead ends and into liberated and unhindered communion.

This freedom requires an effort on my part. Right now it is harder for me to consciously breathe unassisted than to have oxygen delivered into my nostrils. But the nurses keep telling me that what is difficult now is exactly what is necessary to enable me to carry on everyday activities later without getting short of breath. In the same way, it takes more effort to discipline my spirit in prayer and feasting upon God's Word than to be a spiritual couch-potato and passive consumer of random religious blessing.

Jesus has freed me so that I can walk toward Christ and offer myself as a living sacrifice in service to my Lord and Savior (Rom. 12:1).

108 ❧

Good News Travels Fast

DAY 3 IN THE HOSPITAL has been busy with doctors' visits and a few friends coming in shifts, arranged by Andy so he could get to work for a few hours.

There is good news. Dr. Straznicka has seen a preliminary report and had a conversation with the pathologist. She says she took out every lymph node she could get her hands on, and every single one has come back negative, clear of cancer. The tumor, which was safely encapsulated within the lung lobe, has been examined under a microscope, and it's dead. The Beast is slain and banished; 99.5 percent of the tumor cells are necrotic, and the entire thing is safely out of my body.

The surgeon has talked with my oncologist, and the question now on the table is whether I need round four of chemo. My oncologist is the biggest skeptic of the bunch, so if she says, nah, you don't need it, I will take her word for it. We have six weeks to decide.

Just to demonstrate how good news travels, I have had visits today from three *other* docs in this oncology practice, all of whom have heard the good news and wanted to congratulate me. I'm thrilled they are all reading this development as a clear win, but I am not the one to be congratulated. God is the one to be thanked, and I do so with a full heart— even if we decide to do more chemo.

109 &

Pain Management—Part 2

YESTERDAY THE SURGEON INTRODUCED AN interesting exercise. She said, "Okay, now if you need something for pain, you have to ask for it. We have to get you ready to go home, able to manage things on your own."

Until then I had not experienced pain past maybe a 4 (on a scale of 1 to 10). What I was feeling could be more accurately described as discomfort. Yesterday progressed nicely, but by this morning I was feeling an upswing of that internal torso pain that had been masked by medication all week. So for the first time, I requested pain meds because I was finally face to face with the real thing. It turns out I needed only one more dose of the good stuff, and then we devised a plan that will enable me to go home late today. My nurses have been so great, so responsive to my participation in decisions related to my care.

Some spiritual parallels to this pain experience are worth considering. Many of us endure chronic pain of one kind or another: grief, heartache, psychological pain caused by abuse or abandonment, fear that God has it out for us, or chronic physical pain. We may become highly skilled at medicating ourselves with a slow drip of alcohol, Valium, or other anesthetizing substances. We may avoid ever being alone. We may keep the music playing, the television on, or the computer humming. If we were to unhook ourselves from these props, we might discover that coping with pain in the silence or inactivity is impossible.

There is an upside to pain, however. Years ago I had a severe back spasm that had me flat on the floor for ten days. It was the residual pain that instructed me in new body mechanics—if that stretch hurts, find another position for that reach. Yes, it is humane and compassionate to alleviate pain, but not without addressing the root problem causing it. Pain draws attention to what is broken.

I believe God allows pain to break through so its underlying cause can get our attention and move us to seek help. God knows it isn't just the pain that is the problem. It is helpful to think of pain—especially psychological and emotional pain—as a messenger of the brokenness, or perhaps even sin, that is crying out for healing or forgiveness. God allows the pain to continue long enough for us to realize our deep need for his presence and power, moving us to ask him for strength and release from the spasms of bad circumstances, our spiritual rebellion, or the world's injustices. Then we can heal under the lovely ministrations of "the balm of Gilead" (Jer. 8:22).

The psalmist understood this concept well. In Psalm 32 David observed that as long as he withheld confession of his sin, he withered. But when he admitted his guilt, he was restored. In Psalm 13, David lamented his soul-pain and sorrow, and God met him with steadfast love and generosity. The message here is, "Don't suffer needlessly! Ask for pain relief, and submit to healing where things are really broken! God will help you!" Along the road to recovery—a *long* road, especially in grief or mental illness or chronic physical conditions—may the Lord surround us all with loving people with whom it is safe to say, "I am hurting because of [this]. Will you pray for me?"

110 ✍

Making the Transition Home

THURSDAY, MARCH 6, 2014, 4 P.M.

I WILL BE LEAVING THE hospital in an hour or two. It took a while, but I have finally received the okay from respiratory therapist, surgeon, and oncologist. I'm still anemic, compounding my postsurgical fatigue, so my pace is going to be slow and easy for a while. Doc's goodbye instructions are "no flying, no scuba diving, no high-altitude hiking for a month"—like I am so tempted to do those things right now. I want to manage my pain wisely and effectively while working out a plan for reconditioning my body.

Aunt Wendy is driving up from Santa Barbara as we speak, so I will have good help these first few days. Andy says we are having filet mignon for dinner. Why not celebrate with a blood-building steak? I am so grateful for the many ways God has showed his mercy.

111 🌿

Managing Postoperative Discomfort

FRIDAY, MARCH 7, 2014

DAY FIVE POST-OP: MY CHALLENGE today is figuring out how to get and stay comfortable at home. We do not have a high-tech hospital bed that adjusts to the right height and angle, so it took a couple hours to get settled down for sleep last night. I did manage to sleep from midnight to 6:00 a.m., which is the longest span all week.

I'm uncomfortable, in some pain, coughing, and dealing with continued drainage from the surgical site. Bleh. I get up and walk around periodically, position myself with a "coughing pillow" to brace for those deep, muscular, productive heaves of phlegm. It's all normal, but certainly not on my fun list. Aunt Wendy is keeping an eye on my surgical dressing and doing everything else for me, including shopping for tonight's dinner.

All I can do right now is curl up in my recliner and do those infernal breathing exercises. Relying on God that this phase will pass quickly, that I won't lose my sense of well-being, that I use wisdom throughout the day, and that I keep a joyful heart.

112

What a Difference a Day Makes

SATURDAY, MARCH 8, 2014

YESTERDAY WAS PROBABLY MY LOWEST point, but after a particularly restful night, I awoke today feeling much more alert and hopeful.

My little breathing machine (an "inspired volume" measurer) is my friend, indicating that my lungs are opening up more. Respiratory exercises will be the key to continued pulmonary improvement, less light-headedness, and more brain power.

My goal today is to sing a song at the piano without passing out.

I also think I will double the length of my outdoor walk and tour our entire half-acre lot front to back.

Overnight, I have reduced pain meds. All in all, I feel like I am on the mend now.

I am humbled by the success of the treatment and trust God will be showing me how to use my time and talents for his glory.

113 ✑

Progress One Step At a Time

TUESDAY, MARCH 18, 2014, 9 A.M.

TWO WEEKS AFTER LUNG SURGERY, I can detect some slight improvement in my stamina, stair climbing, and breathing. It's a good sign
when I assemble a to-do list and actually accomplish it. Still, twinges of
pain and that pesky fatigue linger, making my days feel long and, yes,
boring. I am getting antsy for progress.

My husband emailed me earlier today with confirmation of our Yosemite wilderness permit. The plan is to hike to the top of Half Dome
over Labor Day weekend. Whether a step of faith or folly, this permit certainly sets a goal out there for me. I have made one unsuccessful attempt
of the Rock and—knowing how hard it is—truly wonder if I can be in
peak physical condition six months after surgery and maybe four months
after round four of chemo yet to come.

So far the only guidance I have from the surgeon about physical activity is "no flying, no scuba diving, and no high-altitude hiking for one
month." Otherwise, the word has been "listen to your body and do what
you feel like doing." Right now my body is saying, "Stay in the recliner."
Inertia is powerful, so I need to find a way to progress in fitness before I
fritter away a perfectly good six months of exercise to meet my Yosemite
goal.

Goal setting plays a role in spiritual fitness too. I occasionally encounter individuals who express a desire to be spiritually fit and immune
to tribulation, close to God, and perfect in every way. (They might not

put it exactly that way, but that's what they are thinking.) They admire Mother Teresa and wish they could be like her but have no idea what it takes to become a saint. With only an impossible dream that saddles them with guilt, they cannot identify a means for getting from Point A—today's disappointing spiritual life—to Point B, that idealized vision of life in Christ.

There is no one-size-fits-all formula or rigid timetable for spiritual growth. We know from Scripture and the witness of many saints throughout Christian history that spiritual maturity is the result of an intentional, lifelong commitment to baby steps. One will not see progress within a week's time, but it is possible to see development month by month. The daily increments of improvement are small, but they eventually add up to a life that mirrors that of Jesus Christ, a person living for the sake of others.

During my convalescence I have been reading a marvelous book by Thomas Ashbrook called *Mansions of the Heart*.[17] The author unpacks the seminal work of Teresa of Ávila (1515–1582) titled *The Interior Castle*. This sixteenth-century Spanish mystic endeavored to describe her soul's journey toward God. Her extended metaphor describes sanctification as a journey through seven "mansions" toward the center of the castle, where communion with Christ is complete. Like tourists wandering through the unfamiliar corridors of a large estate, we faith seekers sometimes go in circles spiritually. But if we cooperate with the Holy Spirit, who is leading us toward the center where "the joyful Trinity" resides, we can know the love of God and experience the true freedom of his righteousness.

Many people take the opportunity during Lent to practice disciplines or self-denial in order to grow in faith and spiritual fitness. I have chosen this year to engage with the ideas Saint Teresa expounded and Dr. Ashbrook explained. By doing so I hope to become more aware of incremental spiritual progress, find encouragement in that growth, and apply the benefits of spiritual fitness and strength not only to my cancer season but also to the day-by-day demands we all face.

---

[17] The conceptual framework of entries March 19–April 2 is provided by R. Thomas Ashbrook, *Mansions of the Heart: Exploring the Seven Stages of Spiritual Growth* (San Francisco: Jossey-Bass, 2009). Used by permission of the author.

114 &

Two-Week Post-Op Checkup

Tuesday, March 18, 2014, 7 p.m.

I SAW THE SURGEON Dr. Straznicka late this afternoon to remove the two sutures and to check me over. Lungs sounded perfectly clear to her. I brought a list of questions, which she answered:

What is this pain in localized spots? "It's inevitable that we tweak some nerves during surgery, and it takes a few weeks for them to settle down. There's no problem exercising around the pain. You won't hurt anything." Okay, I can live with that; it's really just discomfort.

Why am I wheezing upon exertion? "It's normal at this stage, but if wheezing is still an issue four weeks from now, it would time to consult a pulmonologist. However, your lungs are clear, so it's probably a bronchial tightening, to be expected as things move around in there to make up for the lost lung lobe." Using my asthma inhaler might help, and maybe a humidifier too. She also recommends pulmonary rehab. Most people in pulmonary rehab classes, she said, are far worse off than I, even dependent on oxygen. But *everybody* benefits from this program, and it can hasten my recovery.

Can I go backpacking next summer? Andy has acquired for us a Yosemite wilderness permit to climb Half Dome in Yosemite National Park on Labor Day weekend. How do you feel about that? "Great. You should be ready by then. Six months out? No problem. Bring in a picture!"

How about carrying a thirty-pound pack? "The weight won't be a particular issue, but you probably will need some extra padding on the Vein Access Port (VAP) site to protect the skin from a blister. Otherwise, train up for it."

When can I start working out at the gym? "Now. Start easy so you don't strain yourself after so many months off. But progress as fast as your body lets you; it's good for you. You won't faint; you'll know when to stop."

When do I see you again? "In four weeks; one more post-op checkup. Then the next time will be when we take out the VAP."

Dr. Straznicka weighed in on the advisability of going round 4 in chemo. She said, "If you were my mother, I'd tell you go for it. You tolerated chemo so well, and it really worked. You have nothing to lose and everything to gain by that extra insurance." So I think that is decided. By the way, she said, "All indications are that you are cured." How good is that?

I am so encouraged! I floated through my thirty-minute walk, finally finding an aerobic pace. I will find that happy spot again tomorrow and see how much longer I can go.

Tomorrow morning I have my post-op checkup with the oncologist. I hope to have a date for chemo round 4, so I can do a little planning.

115 ✧

Round Four of Chemo Scheduled

ANDY AND I HAD HALF an hour with Dr. Chen this morning. As a result, we have a better sense of what the next several weeks will involve.

We decided to go ahead with a fourth round of chemo and scheduled it to begin Monday, April 21 (the day after Easter), and conclude Monday, April 28. This will be an exact replica of previous rounds—a precaution because of the few viable cancer cells in the tumor that was removed. I am grateful that Dr. Chen was open to timing that preserves my freedom to worship and serve during Holy Week and on Easter morning.

Once chemo is done, the medical surveillance schedule requires a CT scan and physical exam every three months for two or three years, then scans every six months until the end of the fifth year. Dr. Chen's vigilance is directed toward any signs of swollen lymph nodes, errant blood counts, lung nodules, or metastasis (cancer appearing in other organs of the body).

Dr. Chen strongly urged me to get into pulmonary rehabilitation as soon as possible, to maximize my breathing and boost my chances of accomplishing an ascent of Half Dome on Labor Day. I was so discouraged later in the day when I called the pulmonary rehab center for an appointment and was told they cannot even schedule an intake interview for two months!

116 ✍

An Answer to Prayer

THURSDAY, MARCH 20, 2014

YESTERDAY'S NEWS THAT I WOULD have to wait until mid-May for an interview with the pulmonary rehab facility had me down in the dumps. But guess what? Late in the day, my "home visitor"—a church member whom I had never met but who had signed up on "Mary's Helping Hands"—came over after reading my prayer request for a solution to the pulmonary rehab delay. She revealed that she is a respiratory therapist! She said, "I can come over a couple times a week and work with you until you can get into the program!" She gave me my first breathing exercise and directed me to purchase a "spacer" that would make my inhaler work better. We both saw our meeting as a God-thing—definitely an encouragement.

Also, this morning I went to the gym for the first time in almost five months. I did fifteen minutes on the treadmill (2.5 mph, maintaining a heart rate of 105), ten crunches, and seven push-ups. Gotta start somewhere! But I did it!

117 🍃

A New Daily Routine

MONDAY, MARCH 24, 2014

My God-sent respiratory therapist is putting me through my paces.

Now firmly regimented, my days are organized around three daily sessions of respiratory exercises, breathing measurements, and pitifully slow walks, during which I am required to maintain a 95–99 percent oxygenation level. The goal is to be able to walk for six minutes; today, on my first try, I couldn't maintain the oxygen level for more than a minute and a half at a time.

My new friends: a pulse oximeter (measures oxygen in the blood), a peak flow meter (measures breathing function), and an albuterol inhaler with spacer (to open my airways). I feel like a newborn fresh out of the womb learning how to breathe. My RT assures me that at three weeks post-op, I am running races around other lung patients. Not that it's a competition or anything.

Before this new discipline was introduced, I had been increasing my walking pace and even trying some hills. Now the discipline is to build stamina without getting to the point of being out of breath. That means maintaining a heart rate of no more than 110 while keeping my oxygenation above 92 percent. This is no mean feat.

Allergy season and asthma are making my wheezing worse, so we're also working on breathing techniques and relaxation to keep panicky response from setting in. It is so mental, but fascinating, especially considering how helpful my vocal training is turning out to be.

My personal RT is fun, and she explains things really well. Today she said, "Remember, you are only three weeks out from surgery. You're doing great!" Once again, through other people, the Lord is building patience in me.

118 ✑

Teresa of Ávila: New Life in Christ

THIS LENT IS UNLIKE ANY other I have ever experienced. The usual approach for me is to embark on a six-week spiritual examination, perhaps on a theme, often focused on breaking bad habits or confronting spiritual counterfeits in my life. This year I am looking back on my life to identify missteps, detours, and regrets—while I still have some time to make them right, if necessary.

A few weeks ago, not sure whether I would live or die, I started taking stock of my life and wondering if my spiritual goals have been well placed. In previous seasons of self-evaluation, I have used various images to describe my progress in the Christian life. One of my favorites was the spiritual roadmap, in which I drew a map of my spiritual journey. The descriptive exercise was important for observing how and when God had acted to transform me and get me in touch with my soul. I tracked periods of rapid growth (depicted by freeways), spiritual aridity (a desert), special retreats (mountaintops), and even depression (a deep hole). I would depict my current moment as an oasis—a place to stop, rest, recover, and breathe deeply.

The desire to observe the spiritual life is nothing new. St. Augustine's fifth-century spiritual memoir *Confessions* is classic; more recently, in the twentieth century, Thomas Merton chronicled his "journey to peace" in *The Seven Storey Mountain*. Teresa of Ávila employed the stages, or dwelling places, of her journey toward God as a teaching tool for others seeking intimacy with God. When I first read her *Interior Castle* as a seminary student, I got about halfway through it. She was writing about spiritual experiences I had never had and using terms I could not comprehend. Her ardor was unimaginable to me, so I put it aside and wrote an honest book report for class: Help! I have no idea what this woman is talking about. I have not picked it up since—that is, until this week.

While even Teresa eventually found its later stages difficult to put into words, she used the governing image of a castle comprising seven "mansions" to describe her spiritual progression. We would probably call these mansions "rooms." The first step begins at the front door, and each successive room gets closer and closer to the very center of the castle. Passing from one mansion to the next illustrates growth into a new level of spiritual awareness, practice, and relationship with God. Each area is characterized by particular spiritual disciplines, prayer patterns, and attacks by the Evil One, who is hell-bent on us *not* getting to the center place of intimate communion with God.

The first room is found right inside the front door of the castle. I recall when I was first introduced to Jesus—when I first became aware that Jesus was not only Lord and Savior but also Shepherd of *my* soul—it involved stepping out of "the world without Christ" and into a new relationship made possible by Christ's salvation that brought me alive spiritually (Eph. 2:7–10). My first steps were tentative, and I was tempted to second-guess the value of life in Christ. I even kept the front door ajar for a quick escape if needed.

I stepped into the foyer of the interior castle when I was seventeen years old. God providentially placed me in the context of the Catholic charismatic movement sweeping through Seattle in 1970. It was at a "charismatic inquiry night" that I heard the gospel proclaimed, but it took several months for me to give up my pride and summon the courage to actually step into a new life in Christ. The immediate evidence that something serious and life changing was happening to me was an irrepressible joy and a voracious appetite for God's Word. I felt lifted above life's mundane circumstances and into a "room" where new music was playing, the voice of Jesus could be heard, power to change was available, and prayers were answered. I knew little about the Bible or even Jesus at this stage but was intent upon learning, and God met me there.

God asked me to repent. I had to turn away from a life characterized by selfishness and pride and ask Jesus to help me forsake unhelpful habits and establish life-giving ones. Even so, my early prayers centered on requests for help and relief amid my typical teen issues. In the midst of this major reorientation of my life, Jesus reassured me that his grace is real and his love for me is great. I realized that he could be trusted.

Now, forty-four years later, new challenges such as lung cancer confront me. It is encouraging to recall those early days of conversion, reorientation, and life change. I continue to give thanks to God for lifting me out of one world—a highly anxious family system that was nurturing narcissism in me—into God's realm of tender love and reassuring care. I realize that I would have become an entirely different person if Christ had not captured me then. But he did, and I rejoice that this was the beginning of a journey in discipleship that continues to this day.

119 ✍

The Second Mansion:
Torn between Two Loyalties

MEASURING SPIRITUAL DEVELOPMENT IS VEXING because assessments are so often performance based. But Teresa of Ávila's movement of the soul through the mansions of the interior castle is fundamentally a progression from the active, performance-based spiritual life to the infused, relationship-based phases of life with Christ.

The second mansion, which I have called "torn between two loyalties," is the phase in which a true struggle ensues. If the first mansion is the castle's foyer, the second mansion is the living room with a good view of the front yard. Spiritual life in this place of welcome is more active, but the view of the world outside remains enticing, and memories of the good old days tempt the pilgrim to forsake the path toward full communion with God. As Thomas Ashbrook observes, "We feel like a schizophrenic in the second mansion." On the one hand, we are discovering the joys of life in Jesus and growing in knowledge and grace. On the other hand, we are still sampling the pleasures of a worldly life. We still get affirmation consistent with earthly values and are only beginning to get a sense of God's true kingdom values. The voice of Jesus is becoming more familiar, and he is alerting us to the new choices before us.

Meanwhile, Satan is pushing back. The spiritual battle is fraught with temptation, second-guessing, and dabbles in the old life to see what will happen. The clash of values leaves us feeling hypocritical one moment and abjectly dependent on God the next. This early stage constitutes a tug-of-war for our soul. Perhaps for the first time, the Holy Spirit has made our hearts receptive to God's Word, as he challenges the way we have always done things. Then we have a choice that can be agonizing, especially when it entails forsaking a worldly friend who is big trouble or withstanding the ridicule of unbelievers.

When we pray at this stage, we are responsive to Jesus's voice, though we are still primarily talkative and directive: "Here's what I need and how you can meet it." But prayers at this stage also begin to focus outward as we learn to pray for others' needs.

I went through this room my senior year in high school, after committing my life to Christ the previous summer. My spiritual issues did not revolve around drug use, belligerence, troublemaking, or other observable maladies. I was a straight-A student, active in my church, clean living, a typical firstborn overachiever. What was worldly in my soul was a huge dose of pride and conceit, a need to be applauded. I was driven to be the best at everything in order to boost my own reputation. When Jesus got a grip on my life, I was wrested from center stage and introduced to an entirely different reason for living: to glorify and to serve my heavenly Father. The change in my attitude, from the inside out, was observed and commented upon by my choir acquaintances: "What's happened to you? You're not conceited anymore."

Nevertheless, senior year is senior year. I was taking SATs, accumulating "points" for graduation, starring in *Hello, Dolly!* (talk about center stage), and preparing a valedictorian address. This year was both glorious and stalled, spiritually speaking. God protected me through it and set in motion a series of circumstantial developments that would change my life forever. I drifted between the interior castle and the world, sometimes feeling the tug-of-war between them, sometimes falling for the old lures.

But for the first time I experienced a battle within, and according to Teresa of Ávila, this is progress. Before, I had never resisted Satan's enticement to hog the spotlight. Now Jesus was right there, urging a better way and giving me a taste of humility and generosity of spirit. It meant choosing some new friends. It meant becoming more familiar with biblical language and the realities it unveiled. It meant a major shift in focus from myself at the center to Almighty God at the heart of my life. The process of conversion was underway, but the castle still held more rooms.

120 🖋

The Third Mansion: Following Jesus

MOVING SUCCESSFULLY BEYOND THE TUG-OF-WAR stage of the second mansion means the question of whether I will fully commit to life with this Savior has been settled. When temptations rise or trials unfold, I'm not in danger of running out of the house and back into the world. Not that Satan doesn't try to derail the Christian in the third mansion, but the tactics become maliciously subtle, encouraging the development of pride as a person grows in the disciplined life.

The third mansion is characterized by balance in the spiritual life between Bible study, prayer, church participation, and ministry involvement. It is a period known for its doing, and for many believers it is the most productive and even sustainable phase of their walk with Christ. Ashbrook observes that "ministry is often focused on the requests of others, as well as attempts to meet our own needs." This can come across as driven hustle, as the Christian easily confuses working *for* God as relationship *with* God.[18]

Teresa observed that the church tends to accompany people along the spiritual journey only through the third mansion, after which the path is so personal and intense as to be incomprehensible to others. Spiritual maturity eventually involves degrees or phases of development beyond what the church itself can foster. If we truly desire to become steadfast,

---

[18] Ashbrook, *Mansions*, 98f.

passionate, humble disciples of our Lord Jesus Christ, we are going to fly from the church's nest from time to time. Worship attendance, tithing, and participation in church activities represent hallmarks of an active phase. As the soul moves closer and closer to the center where it meets and communes with "the joyful Trinity immersed in God's love," the church's role, with its emphasis on busyness, can actually thwart spiritual progress. The true signs of spiritual growth, such as a thirst for God, manifest in the inner life of the believer rather than in the outer life of activity. Jesus is wooing us into deeper personal intimacy with him, which we can experience if we allow time for reflection in a busy schedule.

In line with the emphasis on doing in this phase, prayer becomes more structured as we take time to remember and appreciate God's presence and power. Whereas earlier prayer majored in personal requests and intercession, now we are more apt to use something like the well-known ACTS pattern for prayer, starting with Adoration and Confession, moving into Thanksgiving and then Supplication. Moments of thrilling spiritual blessing, like my hammock experience last fall, build faith and expand vision, although these moments are infrequent, even rare. Nevertheless, learning how to listen to Jesus becomes more important. It helps to seek out mentors and teachers who can show us how to pay attention to God's presence and activity within.

The majority of my life has been lived in this room of the castle. I became a fully participatory church member shortly after graduation from college and marriage. Within six months, a staff leader at my church snagged me for an administrative assistant job in its music department. This first exposure to the inner workings of a congregation opened up new opportunities to serve, and gradually I discovered and developed my primary spiritual gifts of teaching and preaching. Seminary studies not only fed my mind but also facilitated deep reflection in my soul, as I experienced inner healing that resulted in a significant spiritual transformation. After several years as a lay specialist in ministry to adults, I was ordained in 1987 to the Presbyterian pastorate. Meanwhile, I was gaining both broad and deep exposure to Scripture, learning how to trust God, acquiring ministry skills, and otherwise aligning my life to God's will and way.

Many churches are thrilled when their parishioners arrive at this stage. Their enthusiasm, commitment, and productivity make them hot commodities in the congregation. Pastors love to recruit them and unleash their talents for the benefit of the church body. As the designer of many a church program in my day, with the overachiever tendencies of my youth still nipping at my heels, not to mention my prowess at engaging just the right person for a particular ministry, I know the temptation to keep people busy with church activity. If it were up to churches and their pastors, they would not allow anyone to grow past this stage, because these are the folks who get the jobs done so worship happens, children are taught, and buildings maintained. This thwarting is not intentional, but we were taught to believe that a growing Christian is a productive one. An active participant is maturing in faith. What Teresa tells us is this: if people are flourishing in this active phase, it is only a matter of time before a certain holy dissatisfaction takes hold and makes them search for something more. A wise counselor will recognize this sign of readiness and usher them into the next mansion.

121 ✑

The Fourth Mansion:
Discovering the Love of Jesus

TUESDAY, MARCH 25, 2014

ONE OF THE SPIRITUAL ACCOMPLISHMENTS of my season of lung cancer has been an exit from the rat race, a transition that has been long in coming, since I left the full-time pastorate in 2006. Various projects kept me busy and overstimulated for another five years: studying for a Doctor of Ministry degree, conducting denominational business, serving on a citizen's committee in my city, and teaching master's-level classes at the seminary. But since 2012 I have been working at home in a virtually self-directed manner, writing and preaching occasionally. Last fall this illness hit, and its treatment modulated my pace down to a slow-motion ride through each day.

This prolonged illness coincides with spiritual development identified by Teresa as the fourth and fifth interior mansions. I am drawing from personal experience when I try to explain the fourth stage, discovering the love of Jesus. Teresa considers it a transitional stage, typified by seeking rather than finding.

What characterizes this stage more than anything is seeking to know and experience the love of Jesus Christ at a deep and profound level. Hunger and thirst for an intimate relationship with our Lord becomes the focus of prayer and ministry. Motivated more by love than obligation, the spiritual search is not to appease a dissatisfied God but to become content, trusting, and calm in the knowledge of God's love. This stage introduces the beginnings of "infused prayer," waiting on God's agenda for our time together, rather than defining it on my own terms.

In 2007 I experienced my first twenty-four-hour silent retreat. The instruction was to put aside my agenda—work, assigned readings, to-do list—and simply live in the moment, observing my surroundings, taking walks, listening for God, contemplating Scripture. Waiting upon the Lord and opening up to the topics God wanted to address in my soul relegated *my* list and *my* agenda to a lower priority. The focus turned to knowing God better by beholding him, much as the psalmist described in Psalm 27:4:

> One thing I asked of the LORD,
>   that will I seek after:
> to live in the house of the LORD
>   all the days of my life,
> to behold the beauty of the LORD,
>   and to inquire in his temple.

Rather than business first, prayer second, the longing in the fourth room is for prayer first, business second. Martin Luther was a model of this priority of soul-feeding prayer. His secretary—assisting him with his translation of the Bible into German while exiled in the Wartburg Castle—was known to have nagged the Reformer for spending too much time in prayer (up to three hours in the early morning) when there was so much urgency to finish the translation. And yet Martin, like so many saints in church history, felt his efforts fueled by his time beholding God's glory and seeking guidance and instruction for the day.

God, meanwhile, is taking the initiative to reveal his glory and goodness, sometimes by simple touches of grace in everyday life. On vacation, our then six-year-old daughter Judy fell head first off the top bunk onto a concrete floor. Parental anxiety mounted on the moonless fifty-mile drive to the nearest hospital. When we arrived at the ER, the admitting nurse looked like the identical twin of a pastor back home. It was as if God were saying, "It's okay; my friends are surrounding you in my love right now." God provided a rock-solid floor for us to stand on and never let us sink into fear or despair after that moment. He carried us through the overnight period of evaluation to the joyful confirmation that Judy's skull had not been broken and her concussion was mild.

As we behold God's glory and holiness in times like this, we feel more acutely the contrast with our own failings and wounds. A characteristic of this stage is our desire to confess sin, deal with old emotional wounds, and otherwise resolve unfinished business requiring our forgiveness or even restitution. I have found the guidance of a spiritual director or Christian therapist to be invaluable, and journaling through the process has helped me clarify thoughts and responses to particular situations.

One of the most profound experiences of my life took place in 2007 while taking a course with Dallas Willard, a University of Southern California professor of philosophy and author on Christian spirituality. During the silent retreat, I was jarringly reminded of a wound going back to when I was five years old. My twenty-seven-year-old mother of three children five and under, at her wits end and in need of a nap, locked me out of the house one afternoon. I sobbed and pounded on the back door, trying to persuade her to let me back in. It is hard to say how long my distress continued, but I later recalled the experience as a motif of the emotional distance that lasted decades between us.

Then fifty years later on retreat, God stepped in to reframe my experience. Along with the very painful memory, I had a glimpse of Jesus on a tree swing nearby, saying to me, "Oh, Mary, it's all right. Don't worry about what your mom is thinking behind that door; come and play with me! I love you and want to be your friend!" Whenever I am tempted to replay the hurt of that day, I go back to this playful, safe, and compassionate Jesus, and he has brought healing and completeness to me in that area. This is fourth mansion work, soaking in the love of God.

The devil is active as always, distracting our quiet times with the Lord or enticing us back into that crazy busyness that crowds our appointments with God. The Evil One would love for us to respond with anxiety, indulgent self-love, or narcissism to the wounds we have incurred. Again, some guidance from a mentor or spiritual director helps keep matters in perspective.

At this stage of my cancer recovery, I feel less need to be the center of my friends' tender ministrations. I have loved their gracious attention and the concern of those who have cooked meals. But as my health improves, I feel the Holy Spirit's prod to wean myself off all this attention, throw my full weight on Christ alone, and find ways to give God's loving attention to others.

The best way to cooperate with God's movement into the fourth mansion is to plan quiet time to detach myself from temporal concerns in order to behold God. Providentially, these few months of feeling like a slug, immobile in a lounging position, have made this detachment much easier. Under normal circumstances, I need some time each day, perhaps a day away per month, and an extended period of silence and solitude at least once a year to loosen my grip on worries and agitation. It takes me several hours to settle down and release the distractions of everyday life, so one day is barely enough to get to that quiet place within. But with practice and discipline, I've developed new skill in relinquishment and quieting of the spirit, aided of course by our gracious Lord, who woos me into his presence for the conversation he looks forward to as well.

122 ✑

The Fifth Mansion:
Longing for Oneness with God

HAVE YOU EVER WONDERED WHAT Jesus was really praying for when he asked his heavenly Father to make us one with Jesus, as Jesus is one with the Father? (John 17:22–23).

The idea of oneness conjures up different images. The Eastern religious view of "oneness with the universe," as I understand it, conceives the goal of life as absorption into the one cosmic being after death. Only that universe remains in existence, all other beings having become part of it. Oneness in this case means the complete assimilation of persons into an all-encompassing being and the loss of their individual identities. The Christian worldview does not espouse this.

Oneness with God in the Christian understanding is a complete and accurate alignment of our life to God's. We still exist and function as distinct individuals, but in Christ our will is lovingly wrapped in and shaped by the will of God, such that we ultimately become "Christlike" (1 John 3:2). The New Testament offers plenty of evidence that we retain our unique personhood. We were each created in the image of God. After we die, we each are judged before the throne, and we each are assigned to either heaven or hell, according to God's sovereign judgment of where we belong. The Book of Revelation points (twice—Rev. 5:10 and 22:5) to the vision of God's people reigning with him, suggesting rather strongly that not only do we retain our individuality but we are also given responsibilities to carry out in the new heaven and new earth. There will always be a "Mary" whose sole purpose is to love God, glorify him forever, and do his bidding according to his purposes. All for God.

So as we approach the fifth mansion in Teresa of Ávila's interior castle, we come with a deepening desire to be so close to Jesus that we cannot be separated by circumstances, competing agendas, or spiritual forces. We do not yet experience this ongoing, ultimate unity with God (that is the hallmark of the seventh mansion), but we *want* it more than anything. Lent, earmarked in the church year for intentional spiritual growth, is a good time to cultivate this desire.

In this fifth mansion, we have fallen in love with Jesus and will do anything to demonstrate our love and loyalty to God by submitting to his central place in our lives. In the power of this spiritual magnet, our service in the Lord's name takes on new effectiveness, often without our realizing it. At this stage, "work has become prayer; prayer has become work, all loving God."[19]

The fifth mansion is not a place I dwell in consistently—a sign of how much work Jesus has yet to do in my life—but I took a turn in it one day a couple of years ago. In the midst of a legal process to adjudicate a controversy facing my denomination, I was to give lengthy testimony as an expert witness in a Presbyterian judicial hearing. I knew it would be stretching and difficult, requiring intense spiritual, emotional, and intellectual effort. God had strongly impressed upon me that this trial was an opportunity to love him with "all [my] heart, mind, soul, and strength; and to love my neighbor" (Mark 12:30). I realized that the legal work leading to this moment had become my expression of love to God in the fullest sense; I brought all I had and put it at God's altar as my prayer. During the hours of testimony I gave that day, I felt as one with God's purposes as I ever have, fully used of him (in the best sense), alive, and in awe of what God was doing in our midst.

Prayer in the fifth mansion takes the form of contemplation leading to "absorption and silence" before God. This is where we become

---

[19] Ashbrook, *Mansions*, 134.

speechless before our Creator, Redeemer, and Sustainer. We are simply in awe of God's beauty and power and deeply grateful for his love. Rather than bringing lists of petitions, we are more apt at this point to hold a person before God for his attentive care, healing, transformation, whatever . . . God knows and loves this person and knows exactly what is needed.

Alongside these experiences of wonder in God's presence, we also find ourselves more in tune than ever with our failings and the sin that so easily entangles us. A holy but persistent discontent overtakes us as we long to do better, to be pure of heart, and to free ourselves from old hurts. During this time God can even "disappear" for a while, showing us how much we need the Lord and how bereft we are without him. God's silence also invites us to trust not in our feelings but in God himself, whether he shows up or not. He allows the devil, meanwhile, to dig away at our weak spots, unearthing the places where spiritual repentance and strengthening are needed.

When we see how we fail and consider how it happened, we learn where we went off track and what would have been the remedy—for next time. These concrete spiritual experiences of longing, lapses, and learning are what God uses to shape us ever more closely into his image. Tough? You bet. Necessary? Absolutely. Survivable? Most certainly! The One ushering us through this mansion is the Shepherd of our souls.

How can we promote the work Christ would like to accomplish within us at this stage? We continue to pray as full participants in this divine conversation. We continue to read and study the Bible, so our experience is always grounded within the boundaries of orthodox Christianity. We continue to meet with other Christians to experience Christ's life in our midst. We seek spiritual counsel from a mentor or spiritual director. And we arrange our life and world to allow for time alone in peace and quiet with God. We do not feel guilty about "wasting time with God," because beholding him and listening, enjoying the intercession of both Jesus and the Holy Spirit (Rom. 8), are fruitful spiritual endeavors, empowering us to serve the Lord and our neighbor with pure love and joy.

123 ✐

The Sixth Mansion (Part 1): Passionate Love for God

MY HUSBAND AND I WERE married two weeks after college graduation and almost four years after meeting. Our courtship had weathered challenges that revealed our true characters. Over the years, our love had grown from square-dance flirtation to solid commitment to passion. The process of loving involved a deeper knowledge of my beloved, an appreciation of his fine qualities, a willingness to submit my life to his care, and a mysterious chemistry that bound us together in intimate communion. This life experience helps me understand what is yet to come for me in relationship with my Lord and Savior.

Teresa of Ávila describes the sixth mansion in terms of passionate love for God. His wooing, as of a groom calling out to his bride, redefines the spiritual relationship. In previous mansions we received God's love as a father's love for his child. In this mansion, Teresa describes the intensity of passion in almost sexual terms. This is simply an extension of the New Testament metaphor of marriage, in which Christ is the bridegroom and the church is his bride (Eph 5:21ff, culminating in the images of Rev 19:7 and 21:2ff).

I am relying on Teresa's description because I have not reached the sixth mansion myself. I have yet to breathe deeply and passionately in

God's embrace. I have yet to lose myself in God's generous possession of me. I have yet to experience full union with Christ. But I do get glimpses of God's passionate love for me through my husband's tender affection.

Having been loved this enthusiastically, Teresa's greatest desire was to pray and contemplate God's wondrous beauty. She was able to detach from possessions and worldly values because they became less important than knowing Jesus.

Cancer treatment has forced me to let go of a lot of things. Hair, for instance. Think of all the time and effort I have spent over the years keeping up appearances. The apostle Paul expressed this sentiment when he wrote: "I have suffered the loss of all things, and count them but rubbish so that I may gain Christ" (Phil. 3:7–11).

In reality, the interest in stuff—food, gadgets, hair, winning, *Mad Men* reruns—drops away as passion for God overtakes all other attachments. O Lord, my mind understands the necessity of letting go of things; but my heart still clings to trinkets. I am so sorry.

In order for me to advance into the sixth mansion, it is important for me to give over prime time in my day to quiet—alone conversation with and contemplation of God. This requires weeding spiritual thorns, courage in decision-making, and humility, as I realize how much of God I do not yet know.

Not that God is holding anything back. According to Teresa, God in this stage continues to make himself known directly and indirectly. Sixth mansion dwellers hear God speak in a familiar voice, experience ecstatic joy at the throne of grace, and glimpse heaven. I have had isolated experiences of hearing God speak to me (not audibly but strongly), even during my current illness. And yet these moments are punctuated by periods—sometimes years—of silence.

It is important to acknowledge how heavily invested the Enemy is in our spiritual derailment, even to the point of counterfeiting God's voice. Recognizing this spiritual danger, Teresa used three tests to verify that her spiritual experiences were from God (see *Mansions*, 181). The evidences that God is speaking are these: 1) the power and authority accompanying God's word results in God's fulfilling it in our experience; 2) "the great quiet left in the soul"—the peace that accompanies recollection and makes one ready to praise God; and 3) a lasting memory of what God said because of the deep impression it made. My experience in prayer on February 3 satisfies this test. God's word to me, "You don't have to pray about healing anymore; I've taken care of that" is, so far, fulfilled in my experience. I immediately felt at peace about my health situation and give God the credit and praise. And its memory made a strong impression upon my spirit that continues to this day.

Maybe I have a toe in the doorway of the sixth mansion after all.

124 ✍

The Sixth Mansion (Part 2):
The Dark Night

Ordinary Christians advancing on the road to spiritual maturity and union with God have times and seasons when God seems absent and unresponsive. Prayer gets us nowhere; it seems our supplication hits the ceiling and falls right back down into our laps. We derive no blessing from worship, no consolation from prayer, no fruit from Bible study. God tests us with the question, "Do you rely on blessing, consolation, and fruit more than you depend on Me?"

God gives us the opportunity to live without those spiritual perks for a time, in order to establish confidence in the presence and power of God as he knows himself to be and for his own sake, not ours. The deeper we travel through the mansions toward the center of the castle, the more spiritual life is about God and the less it is about us. This is progress!

Many Christians find it difficult to talk about what is known as the "dark night." For an intimate look at this spiritual experience, which itself is not a mansion in Teresa of Ávila's *Interior Castle*, we turn to her sixteenth-century contemporary, John of the Cross. He describes a condition of the spiritual life that flummoxes and disturbs the Jesus follower, especially if one does not see it coming or understand its purpose. But even if one does, the experience is sufficiently heart-wrenching—and sometimes long enough—to leave the most advanced saints trembling in desolation.

The first type of dark night involves losing the sense of God's presence and activity. John of the Cross calls this the dark night of the senses. It is not a product of the imagination. God is launching us on a new challenge intended to mature us as disciples by withholding consolation for a time. In my life, the dark night has been the supreme test of my response: anxiety or trust?

Think of it this way: When we were babies, our cries of hunger or diaper-discomfort were heard and swiftly heeded. We were fed or our diapers were changed. Our parents' God-given job was to respond to our needs with such consistency that we would trust them and bond with them as we developed. As we grew older, we were taught how to walk, feed ourselves, and learn at school, while positively reinforced with pats on the back, gold stars on a chart, or a special treat on a Sunday afternoon. If our family was reasonably healthy, our emotional and psychological maturing eventually developed us into stable, self-reliant adults. If our parents succeeded, we absorbed their wisdom and found a way to live consistent with their values. Such children rise up to call their parents blessed.

God loves us even more than our parents do. After our spiritual birth, our heavenly Father shows nurturing love by responding to our needs, pouring out blessing in large and small doses as needed. Over time we accumulate experiences of spiritual touches that build our faith and reduce our anxiety. But in order for us to become mature in Christ, God disabuses us of the notion that following Jesus is about our feelings of comfort or blessing. Ultimately, God wants us to know that our relationship with him does not rise and fall on a sense of blessing, but rests on him alone. And so, in order to test our progress, God hides the blessings for a time in order to reveal the state of our dependencies.

We can find encouragement in knowing that God is doing something active: purifying our souls of those attachments and dependencies on things that cater to our weaknesses. If we are to trust solely in Jesus, we cannot depend on anything or anyone else for security, love, or affirmation. If we are to trust solely in God, we must know what we cannot trust in ourselves. During the dark night of the senses, God withholds the consolations and anything that feeds our spiritual pride, so that our only reason for living is for God's glory.

E. Stanley Jones, a lifelong Methodist missionary in India, suffered a catastrophic stroke in his old age, rendering him paralyzed and almost speechless. One day a bishop who had retired from service in the archdiocese visited him and bemoaned the loss of his staff, the pomp and ceremony of his office, and the authority he had carried. He poured out the grief that was shaking his faith in God. What was he to do? Jones, bedridden, revealed his secret. "The difference [between you and me] is in giving up the innermost self to Jesus." The bishop had been held together by outer props, now removed by retirement. But, Jones reflected, "I need no outer props to hold up my faith, for my faith holds me." Now *that* is a purified soul![20]

We must stifle the tendency to work harder in order to gain the blessings we miss. The dark night of the senses is like a Lenten season of deprivation that God orchestrates and we endure. On the other side of it, we are convinced of and secure in God's love alone.

John of the Cross then speaks of an even deeper level of dark night, the dark night of the soul. This is perhaps more frightening, as it elicits our fear of abandonment, rejection, and despair. It is one thing to feel the rejection of one's mother for an hour or so, as I did at age five. It is quite another to feel abandoned by God for a month or even years. God is seemingly absent, and we are mortified by the true state of our soul and its weaknesses, our propensity to sin, and the hopelessness of our condition without the redeeming work of Christ.

Robert Robinson was converted under the ministry of evangelist George Whitefield in 1755. He became a minister who penned the words of the beloved hymn "Come, Thou Fount of Every Blessing." Late in life, in his own black hole of spiritual depression, Robinson heard a woman sing his hymn, and remarked, "Madame, I am the unhappy man who

---

[20] E. Stanley Jones, *The Divine Yes* (Nashville: Abingdon, 1975), 63.

wrote that hymn many years ago; I would give a thousand worlds, if I had them, if I could feel now what I felt then." His prayer and ours:

> Prone to wander, Lord, I feel it!
> Prone to leave the God I love!
> Here's my heart, O take and seal it,
> Seal it for thy courts above.

Our hunger and thirst for righteousness is met by God's silence for a time, sometimes years, until God feels we have had enough purifying.

We Protestants sometimes have a problem with the concept of "purification," because we believe that our salvation was fully effected by Jesus Christ upon the cross and there is no further price to pay to satisfy God. To be clear, the dark night is not about paying a price, earning grace, or even pleasing God. It is a ruthless dealing with our old nature, which wants to depend on things and people and not on God. If we want to be Christlike, our lives must align with the Father's will. But this alignment means forsaking all the other things we say aren't important but really are. As the writer of Hebrews said, "In your struggle against sin you have not yet resisted to the point of shedding your blood" (Heb. 12:4). Since we have not willingly chosen to resist the sin that so easily entangles us, God—graciously and patiently—purges our souls of their unholy dependencies. Does it hurt? Unspeakably. Will we survive? God knows our hearts and what we can bear. Will it ever end? Not sure. Ask Mother Teresa.

Perhaps the most heartrending example of the dark night of the soul in recent history is provided by Saint Teresa of Calcutta. In the early 1950s God spoke to her and directed her to start a radical mission to the poorest of the poor in Calcutta. She relocated her life and started a new order in its slums. God blessed her with a facility, a cadre of dedicated sisters, and financial support. God's presence with her was tangible, and she was empowered to launch an amazing ministry. After she was fully committed and the work had begun, God seemingly disappeared. Her prayer life went dry, and her soul cried out to the One who had led her into this risky and costly ministry.

The book *Come, Be My Light* chronicles Teresa's fifty-year spiritual torment.[21] Brian Kolodiejchuk, the priest responsible for investigating her life for potential Catholic sainthood, traces her spiritual development by means of correspondence with her spiritual directors and father confessors. Her experience can only be described as excruciating. After twenty-five years of spiritual desolation despite daily Mass and spiritual devotion, something finally made sense to Teresa: God was allowing her to experience the abandonment and despair common among the people she was reaching through her ministry on the streets of Calcutta. Her compassion for them, in Jesus's name, helped her to smile and pour out the love of Jesus. Until her death in 1997, she never again experienced an outpouring of blessing or even a sense that God was with her. She simply kept talking to God in prayer, offering her life as a living sacrifice, not to earn God's favor but simply to love him through cheerful acts of kindness.

About ten years ago, after nine months of sensing that God was setting me up for a new pastoral call, the interview process fell apart and another person was called to the position. I was devastated by the rejection and, even worse, plunged into a hole of spiritual darkness, where I could not perceive the voice of Jesus. Self-doubts overcame me as I cried out for God's comfort and direction. I struggled over the next year to discern God's voice and gain some reassurance that he was still with me. With no insight or feelings to go on, I was groping in the dark. I did what Mother Teresa did: I kept ministering in my current parish, until God directed otherwise. My faith felt blind, but it held.

I wouldn't wish a dark night on anybody, except for the fact that when God does show up again, there is nothing sweeter, more reassuring, or more thrilling than to be face to face once again with the God who never stopped loving me.

---

[21] Mother Teresa, *Come Be My Light: The Private Writings of the "Saint of Calcutta,"* edited with commentary by Brian Kolodiejchuk, MC (New York: Doubleday, 2007).

125 ✌

The Seventh Mansion: Union with the Trinity

WEDNESDAY, APRIL 2, 2014

IF THE FIRST MANSION WAS the foyer of the castle, the seventh mansion is the safe room at the very center. Arrival here is to have survived the dark nights, the divided loyalties, and the mountaintop ecstasies of faith. The seventh mansion represents the culmination of our spiritual quest, our access to the very heart of God as Father, Son, and Spirit. Entry into the presence of our Savior is to finally experience the Christian life as a normal, (almost) uncontested, and natural way to live. It's like a driver after twenty years behind the wheel: actions and responses are instinctive and second nature.

So it is in the spiritual life. Someday life with Christ is going to be as free and natural as breathing. Yes, I aspire to this ease, considering my current condition four weeks after lung surgery. Breathing does not come effortlessly, wheezing reminds me daily of my constricted airways, and my body is not getting quite enough oxygen. I practice deep breathing, to maximize the airflow and develop greater lung capacity. What a metaphor for Christian discipleship!

Pursuing Teresa's image, we enter the seventh mansion by way of three experiences that never leave us:

- Delightful vision of the Trinity—undistracted by its paradoxes—and welcome into the eternal party of Father, Son, and Spirit.
- Beholding Jesus in his full humanity, similar to the way his disciples encountered him after his resurrection.
- Irresistible oneness with Christ, like the marriage of kindred spirits. For the rest of our lives we live in an ongoing and deepening relationship of unique union with God.

Teresa advises that the seventh mansion is not a state of continuous euphoria or daily ecstasy. Rather, the seventh mansion is characterized by steady breathing in dynamic rhythm with the heartbeat of God. The tussles are over, our fellowship unhindered. Service to others—fueled by the continuous infusion of God's power—is effective and selfless. We experience the freedom that comes from unconditional surrender to Jesus, abandoning ourselves to God.

Previously I found Dallas Willard's description of this dynamic hard to understand, but now I get it. Willard said the goal of the Christian life is such union with Christ that we are free to do what we want. Being the Calvinist I am, with a deep mistrust of my own "totally depraved" instincts, I was mystified by this vision. But Willard's point was, when you are in communion with the Lord, God's will becomes your will, and you experience the freedom Adam and Eve had before the fall to naturally (in the Spirit) do what Jesus would do if he were in your shoes. Since he is, you can!

Prayer at this stage is a continuous, trusting silence before God, "an adoring attentiveness to the Holy Trinity."[22] In this silence we experience full union with the Trinity and a sense that their prayer becomes our prayer. The apostle Paul notes in Romans 8 that both the Holy Spirit and Jesus himself intercede for us with the Father. We simply enter into their prayer life and are transformed by it. This state of continual prayer is sustained by God's loving touches that draw our attention to him and keep us in his rhythm. It is also fueled by extended times of solitude and silence.

---

[22] Ashbrook, *Mansions*, 204.

Prayer such as this keeps us in the present moment, where God is sufficient and gracious and powerful. With this kind of security, the satanic Enemy—try as it might—cannot get our full attention and is repulsed. With God's help we remain vigilant against self-deception or spiritual pride. Accountability to the Christian community prevents us from overlooking our neighbor as surely as God's Spirit keeps our hearts in union with Christ. Within this balance we are empowered to translate the great blessing from God into blessing for others in day-to-day ministry.

This path through the seven mansions of the interior castle has both stretched and encouraged my faith. While my body underwent testing and treatment for disease, God's Spirit searched me and knew my heart. I am thankful for the lens of Teresa's insight into spiritual growth and trust that I am following the path toward communion with our Savior.

Lord, draw us ever closer to your heart, and show us your true, triune nature!

126 🌿

Lenten Loss

ON SATURDAY AFTERNOON MY BROTHER called to say that Mom had suffered a stroke and that I should come right away. Andy and I dropped everything and flew up to Seattle to be with her. She was unconscious by the time we arrived, suffering the effects of a catastrophic brain-bleed. As a family we followed her wishes, imparted in her advance directive for health care; we withdrew life support and switched her protocol to "comfort care." She slipped from this life to the next early yesterday morning.

My sister Martha and I are camping out in Mom's apartment, reminiscing over photo albums, and planning next steps. Brother Mike, who lives locally, is the executor of Mom's estate. Sister Louise is glad for the company of her grown kids while processing her own distanced relationship with Mom. Relatives have been notified that a Mass of the Resurrection will be held next Monday, the beginning of Holy Week. We expect some company, including the arrival of a cousin who is the family's historian.

Through the daze of grief, I am feeling lost emotionally and "off" physically, having lost a lot of sleep and temporarily abandoned my pulmonary rehab regimen. Breathing in this damp Seattle weather has been difficult. Today, circumstances are calmer and more under my control, so I'm hoping to get my personal routines back in place. There is some time pressure to get Mom's apartment emptied and divested, but that will have to wait until I am over round four of chemo and have the stamina to tackle it, probably in June.

It feels too early to reflect on Mom's life and legacy. It's complicated, as mother-daughter relationships are prone to be. But for now I am comforted by the psalmist's observation: "precious in God's sight is the death of his saints" (Ps. 116:15).

127 🖋

Maundy Thursday Reflection

A CONCERN VOICED FREQUENTLY BY dying parishioners and hospital patients I visit goes something like this: "I am not as concerned about my death as I am worried about the grief and adjustments my [husband, kids, coworkers . . .] will experience when I am gone." When this thought is shared with family members, their reactions vary:

> *Denial*—"Oh, don't worry about us, Mom. We'll be fine."
> *Practical*—"Mom, you better give us the passcodes to your devices and accounts, so we can deal with your finances later."
> *Deflection*—"No, no, don't talk like that. We're here together now. That's all that's important."
> *Silence*—". . ."

Jesus dropped hints for months prior to his arrest and crucifixion that he would be leaving his disciples. The gospel writers do not record specific reactions to his predictions, but more often than not, Jesus's followers changed the subject with new questions. What he was saying did not jibe with their understanding of the awaited Messiah, who would reign victoriously over the nation of Israel and bring peace to the land and chosen people. Trial? Death? Rebuild "this temple" in three days? Jesus's references to his death only confused them.

So the night before he suffered and died, Jesus had a lengthy, symbolic dinner with his disciples. He wanted to prepare them for his cruel departure and instruct them for life after his death. John 13 through 17 records Jesus's remarkable demonstration of servanthood, his institution of Communion ("Do this in remembrance of me"), and his reassuring instruction regarding the ministry of the Holy Spirit in his absence. The whole evening was intended to be memorable and preparatory for these dear men who had accompanied him for three years.

I have thought about what I would say to my dear husband, precious daughters, and beloved colleagues right before my death. My loved ones will probably remember whatever I utter for a long time. What will be on my lips?

I want to tell them how much I love them, how capable they all are of living and flourishing without me, and how good God is. I want to remind them of where I am going, by virtue of my trust in Jesus's promised salvation. And I want them to know that in my absence God will comfort and guide them in wisdom, compassion, and hope.

I wish I had some last words from my mother.

128 ✑

Good Friday Reflection

A S I WAS SITTING IN the choir tonight, contemplating the Scriptures, the songs, and the choral pieces offered during our Good Friday service, something struck me forcefully. All four gospel accounts record that Jesus remained conscious throughout his crucifixion ordeal. We know he remained alert because, in each account, he said something right before he died and then "he gave up his spirit" (Matt. 27:50, John 19:30) or "breathed his last" (Mark 15:37 and Luke 23:46).

Jesus was in agony. He was slowly dying of asphyxiation, caused by the unnatural position of his body hanging by the wrists on a cross. The tightness in my chest these days—due to asthma or reactive airways after lung surgery—is nothing compared to the heaviness Jesus felt trying to keep his lungs filled with air. He remained awake and alert while the weight of his body slowly compressed his lungs. This fact alone convinces me that Jesus endured the cross intentionally and rationally. He chose to remain awake: to feel every pain, gasp every breath, and say every word that needed to be said, until, finally, it was finished.

Today this type of death by slow, conscious suffocation, is so rare as to be beyond ordinary experience. In this country, at least, if one is under any kind of medical care at all, the symptoms and side effects of impending death are addressed through pain control, anti-anxiety medications, warm bedding, and supplemental oxygen. Within three hours of the splitting headache that caused her neighbor to call 9–1–1, my mother was unconscious and paralyzed from her stroke. No longer in pain, experiencing no agitation, and aided in breathing by a ventilator, she was accompanied by the kindness of family members keeping watch and nurses ministering their wonders of care and comfort. She slipped into heaven about sixty hours after the initial symptoms set in, and her four children were glad she did not suffer.

But Jesus suffered mightily when he died for us. He missed nothing of the indignity, the agony, and the heaviness of his burden. He carried us and bore our wounds upon himself, and that is why we call Good Friday *good*. He poured out his love for us by taking upon himself what we deserve for our sin. And he did it the hard way.

While I experience as yet unresolved breathing difficulties, while I go back into the chemo cave (on Monday) to feel that cellular-level fatigue, while I fully heal from the amazing surgery that has rendered me cancer free, I want to remember Jesus's painful process that led to my new life. Though I have tried to imagine what he went through, even with my persistent shortness of breath I will never fully know the extent of his resolve. I will only enjoy its benefits.

If I am ever called upon to suffer for the sake of Christ or in service to others, may I do so with eyes wide open, alert not only to the pain but also to its purpose, just as Jesus did.

129 ✑

Pre-chemo Check-In

MY FOURTH AND LAST CHEMO cycle begins the day after Easter. For the last two days—alongside the spiritual experiences of Holy Week—I have had a flurry of medical appointments in preparation.

Dr. Rahman discharged me from her care on Thursday. She has been monitoring the effects of 45-Gray of radiation, which have completely subsided now and are no cause for concern. My skin has healed, my esophagus functions without residual effect, and the upper left lobe, the most beat up by radiation, has been surgically removed. Reflecting on the fine outcome of this treatment, I expressed my delight and gratitude.

Dr. Rahman teared up and reached for a tissue, saying, "Mary, I know your faith made a big difference, not only in your outlook, but in the outcome."

Dr. Straznicka also signed off, declaring me sufficiently healed from surgery to begin chemo. She is a bit concerned that my bronchi are still constricted, causing some wheezing. My four remaining lung lobes are fully inflated now, but my discomfort in breathing needs some attention. Dr. Straznicka prescribed a visit to Dr. Kristina Kramer, pulmonologist, who is booked through the middle of June.

Oncology nurse practitioner Eloise checked over my blood work, which for the most part is normal. My red cell count has risen from 8 to 11.8 in a month but is still below the normal of at least 13. I no longer have to take all that iron each day but will revisit this after I am done with chemo.

Respiratory therapist Cindy examined my peak flow chart carefully and concluded that less-than-optimal breathing is now impeding my progress. By this time I should have had a breakthrough and seen some higher numbers that measure airflow. Instead, the numbers have gone down slightly or plateaued. I was probably too sedentary the last two weeks in Seattle and failed to keep up with my breathing exercises. Now they make me cough and my chest tighten—another reason to get in to see a pulmonologist ASAP. Cindy says "there's a med for that." If so, I sure don't want to wait until June to get it.

The third major treatment of my lung cancer was to remove the affected upper left lobe of my lung, which encased the dead tumor. Last Thursday, my surgeon declared me sufficiently recovered from that operation to proceed to my final precautionary round of chemo, which starts tomorrow. However, I am also dealing with a lingering condition requiring the attention of a pulmonary specialist. The symptoms—tight chest, constricted airways, wheezy breathing—mimic asthma, though it is not clear that this is the cause. Because exercise now causes counterproductive coughing jags, I am stalled in my rehab. We're getting a handle on this now, and a new med is on the way. Things get so complicated when you have four doctors treating you for the variety of medical side effects and clinical conditions that create the cancer constellation.

130 ✑

Feelings and the Christian Experience

Easter Sunday, April 20, 2014

THE CHURCH HAS JUST BEEN through the lows and highs of the Christian calendar, walking with Jesus through his passion and death on Good Friday, experiencing the emptiness of Holy Saturday and the exultation of Easter. Reactions to this emotional ride vary from indifference to obsession, but the intensity of the calendar's events is intended to draw us into Christ's experience in order to appreciate all the more what he did for us.

It is for those who feel almost nothing, though they would like to, that I would like to share my recent experience. I walked through the last week emotionally cautious for a different reason: to get emotional would have exacerbated the physical condition I am struggling with at the moment.

I found out the hard way, as I sat at my dying mother's ICU bedside two weeks ago, that crying causes increased constriction in my chest, uncontrollable coughing, and hyperventilation. I had to leave the room in order, literally, to catch my breath. So crying was not available as an emotional release or an expression of my feelings at such a precious time. As a ministering professional, I have preached or sung at enough memorial services to have learned how to keep my emotions in check. In this case, it was a matter of medical necessity.

And then Holy Week happened, and I was faced with the elation of the triumphal entry into Jerusalem, the depths of Christ's passion and crucifixion, the glory of Easter. And all I could do was go through the motions. I didn't even go to my favorite service of the year on Maundy Thursday. Good Friday carried with it enough distractions (doctors' appointments, picking up a daughter from airport) to keep me on an even keel. I did sing some beautiful choral pieces Friday night, but I could stay in professional mode. And then on Easter morning, we got up early to attend worship at 8:00. It was wonderful, by all objective standards, but because I had not really felt the lows of Holy Week, the highs had far less impact on me.

This situation is common—albeit for a host of different reasons—to many people at this time of year. We ask, "What is wrong with us that we do not feel Easter's impact?" There are several possible reasons: negative associations with anything church related, previous trauma, an addictive habit that has masked pain for a long time, or lives that are too busy to have room for genuine emotion.

But here is the good news: the fact that we don't feel anything does not change the effectiveness of what Jesus did for us two thousand years ago and what God continues to do today. Our gracious God does not require our feelings—or even our faith if you want to get down to it—to do his thing. That thing is redemption: the reclaiming of what is his and its restoration to its proper place within his kingdom. Our emotions (or lack thereof) affect our spiritual *experience* but not the reality of what God has accomplished.

And so, in keeping with the ideas of St. John of the Cross and his dark night of the senses, I am content to place myself in silent readiness for God's touch at the right moment. That place of readiness might be an hour in the porch swing on a spring day, quiet reading of the day's lectionary Scriptures at the kitchen table, or a walk on the beach, listening to God's immense power crash in the waves. Can you find a place of quiet where God can meet you? He won't make you cry if you can't or don't want to. He will simply say, "I did this for you, because I love you."

EASTERTIDE

131 ✍

God Is on the Move Again

ROUND FOUR OF CHEMO IS going to go much easier than previous rounds. Yesterday's long chemo session went without a hitch, and after a couple hours of sleepiness, I was able to move around a bit. I did awake at 3:30 a.m., perky and ready to start the day, which is a chemo-related pattern. But it enables me to write.

My primary care physician came through with a prescription for a corticosteroid yesterday. I feel more hope for a solution to my bronchial discomfort.

Yet another evidence of answered prayer: I called the pulmonologist this afternoon to officially ask for an appointment as soon as possible. The nurse put me on hold, and the word came back that, due to a cancellation, I can go in at noon tomorrow.

Though it is understandable at this stage of chemo, I lament that I am doing no exercise. Last week my workout sent me into a coughing tizzy, which scared me a little. But it's time to get serious about reconditioning, somehow. I think it means going back several workout levels and building up from there. It's humiliating—not that I'm proud or anything—to be exhausted by the silliest little exercises.

132 ✐

Death and Resurrection

"I WANT TO KNOW CHRIST and the power of his resurrection and the sharing of his sufferings by becoming like him in his death." (Phil. 3:10)

So many threads of my life come together in my mother's story, which is now mine to tell and learn from. Over these last few months, I have pondered the meaning of life and death in reference to my own prolonged illness. But now I must process mortality and resurrection in the face of my mother's sudden death.

What I appreciate more deeply from Christ's passion and crucifixion is that Jesus fully understands our sorrow, our pain, and has experienced death itself. What sweet comfort that reality is, and what stupendous hope we have because of his resurrection that followed. The knowledge that our Lord and Shepherd Jesus Christ lives and reigns imparts hope to our entire perspective on life and death.

Coming out of the other side of lung cancer is a sort of resurrection. The forgoing dying has been incremental and spiritual in nature. Now here I am, alive and looking forward to life. What blows me away is that my mom, the one who feared my death most, was the one to die first and unexpectedly, at the end of my cancer journey. Piecing together her story, I believe my illness killed her.

At her funeral, her friends reported to me that Mom was worried sick throughout my illness. She believed the course of my disease would follow that of her brother many years ago; four months after Uncle Bill found out he had lung cancer, he died. I had forgotten (if I ever knew) his cause of death, but his experience offers some explanation for my mother's sudden engagement in my life through those weekly phone calls six months ago. Though she never addressed the subject directly with me, I am quite sure now that Mom assumed I would be dead within four months.

Despite the success of the early treatment, my efforts to provide her with current information about my condition, and the confirmation of "no evidence of disease" after surgery, she could not believe I would live. She obsessed about losing a daughter and was baffled that I was not crippled in fear. Her next-door neighbor quoted Mom as saying, "I just don't think Mary is taking her illness seriously." When I asked how Mom had come to that conclusion, she said, "She felt that you were faking cheeriness and optimism and were in denial about having cancer."

Another friend told me that, despite the postoperative news—all good and celebrated by my doctors—Mom seemed unable to let go of her worry for me. It was one month after my all-clear that she collapsed.

Worrying oneself to death about the life-threatening illness of another is not what Paul had in mind when he described "sharing in Christ's sufferings, becoming like him in his death" (Phil. 3:10). In the school of worry in which I grew up, handwringing was a duty confused with empathy. Worriers feel they are expressing love and care, but they only burden others with the necessity of assuaging the worrier's fears.

I have lived a lifetime aware of my mom's anxiety, and despite her best efforts, her fears became a wedge between us early in my adulthood. By Christmas she had stopped calling weekly, though I called her when news broke. I was so disappointed that these conversations did not open up doors for self-disclosure or heart-to-heart connection, but stayed on a superficial level. To her credit, Mom did not dump her worry on me overtly, and I now know that talking about other things was mostly about helping her feel better. How little I realized how much she needed. I thank God for her friends who tried to give her an emotional outlet and support throughout this period.

But here is what I observe: Worry is done at a distance. Empathy comes close. Worry is isolating. Empathy enters the world of suffering without succumbing to it. Worry spins out in a dead-end cul-de-sac. Empathy carries relationships forward and enriches both sufferer and friend with human dignity. E. Stanley Jones declared, "Worry is atheism," because one cannot harbor fear without losing faith.[23] My mom lived with the tension between worry and faith, and though she was a believer in Jesus Christ, she lost the tug-of-war to worry. This reality is unbearably sad to me.

---

[23] Jones, *Abundant Living*, 74.

133 ✒

Knowing Mother, Knowing Myself

THURSDAY, APRIL 24, 2014

HOW DOES ONE GET TO know one's mother? The question becomes vital as I try to get to know myself.

The process of bonding and understanding begins even before birth and is nurtured early by the intimacy of feeding, bathing, soothing to sleep. The personality types of both mother and daughter are expressed in this dynamic, and a mother's emotional health is a key factor in raising an emotionally stable and secure adult. I did not have that security. I was wounded and tried to compensate for its lack.

My mother was the third and last child in her family, following a biological brother and an adopted sister. She apparently was a surprise baby for whom the family reservoir of emotional energy was empty. Her mother—my grandmother—was herself the product of a large and seriously dysfunctional family. She chose favorites among her children and emotionally abandoned the others. Her children discovered upon her death that she had pitted brother against sister in competition for her affection. She left her estate to only one of the three, thus disinheriting two of her three children; my mom was one of them.

During her childhood, my mother was left to her own devices for emotional stability. She chose to read. She would curl up in the attic for hours at a time with a great book and be transported to another world. We discovered upon perusing her library that she had a particular affinity for Anne Frank. While her older sister was being taught how to cook and sew, Mom was gaining her education through reading. She excelled in school, particularly in history and English, but always felt inferior in math and science and anything requiring spatial reasoning. This translated into serious technophobia as an adult.

She grew up in the 1930s and 40s with the message that she was not particularly loved, appreciated, or worth her mother's time of day. At school, however, her innate intelligence and curiosity were recognized. After particular success in French, she was emboldened to apply to the University of Michigan. She met my dad there, and they were married the summer after her 1952 graduation. My dad gave her the unconditional love and support she needed.

I was born ten months later. By Mom's later account and my own observations, she was immediately in over her head. What new parent isn't? In her case, because she had received so little emotional nurture in her own early life, she did not have a reservoir within herself from which to draw in parenting her children. In order to cover the wounding of emotional abandonment, she began to construct a family system that would protect her fragile center. This meant that her husband and children were required to orbit around her needs. Her limitations became theirs as well, as long as she could persuade them to comply with her demands.

This is perhaps why I have a strong personality. My entire life has been a quest to differentiate myself, to break out of her orbit, and to become the person God designed me to be. Born of two introverts, my gregarious social style was hard for them to handle. I talked too much. I had unrealistic dreams. I liked and excelled in mathematics, while also progressing in music performance. But most of all, I had what are normal emotional needs for nurture and affection, and these were not met in my childhood. In fact, my family system saw those needs as weakness.

With this background, which, I understand, is neither unusual nor unique, it is a miracle of God that Jesus captured my soul when I was seventeen. That was when God began the nurturing and healing process that has by now produced a mature adult. The emotional distance from my parents set the stage for a yearning to be known and loved by God. I am still on the Way. I am grateful to God for bringing my husband into my life. He (and his parents) showed wonderful patience that enabled me to heal. Our two daughters were born before either of us was thirty; I was still undergoing a radical renovation of the heart. Nevertheless, I believe that I have not perpetuated the worst of the previous generation's emotional deficits.

How does one get to know one's mother? Through direct self-disclosure, indirect observation, the reports of family and friends, and perhaps a journal. My mother wrote an autobiography several years ago, and she kept a daily journal for decades. She instructed that her journal be sent to the University of Washington archives, sealed to researchers for fifty years and never open to any of her relatives, ever. I used to feel angry about being denied access, because I have been trying to figure out my mother my whole life.

But now that she is gone, I have one comfort. Because she is known and loved by the One who made her, her story is an open book in heaven. Perhaps I can read it there.

134 🖋

My Mother, Myself, in an
Anxious Climate

FRIDAY, APRIL 25, 2014

MY MOTHER WRITES IN HER autobiography that during her college years she began to experience anxiety, fear, and what was known as scrupulosity, a sort of spiritual obsessive-compulsive disorder. Coming out of a home where the expression of love for her was thin and unconvincing, she was afraid that even God could not love her without serious performance of perfection.

At the same time, she was suffering from clinical anxiety and developing phobias. After a disastrous two-and-a-half-hour tooth extraction when she was twenty, she developed a fear of going to the dentist. To her credit, though, she made sure we four kids had a healthy relationship with dentistry. Mom told me that once, when I was a toddler, the doorbell rang, and she cowered with me behind an inner door until the visitor left.

Mom struggled with anxiety her whole life. Sometimes it was under control; other times it was carried to the point of agoraphobia. Anything could set it off, including a difficult or confrontational conversation.

It wasn't until I left home for college and began interacting with fearless, crazy Stanford classmates that I realized how my mother's anxiety had narrowed my life experiences. The way to deal with anxiety, I learned, was to order your world so thoroughly as to leave nothing to chance. We always knew in advance what we were having for dinner on any given night; where the closest bathroom was; where we would be going to Mass that Sunday (a requirement whenever we were on vacation); and how many hours of sleep we would get.

Consequently, some might have called my lifestyle as a college freshman highly disciplined, but really it was a way of assuaging my inherited anxiety. Up at 5:30 for a quiet time with God, 6:30 grooming, 7:10 breakfast, 7:30 on the bike to get to 8:00 a.m. class. Back to my room for lunch and study all afternoon, dinner promptly at 5:30, and after more studying, to bed by 9:30 p.m. I was a bore of a roommate.

But my greatest anxiety came from attempting to earn the love and respect of my mother. It seemed irreparably lost when I gave my life to Christ the summer between my junior and senior years of high school. After attending a life-changing prayer meeting, I shared with Mom that I was a follower of Jesus—I probably said, "I'm a Jesus-person now."

She laughed in disbelief and walked out of the room, unwilling to talk about it. She thought it was a phase I would grow out of. She certainly had no category within her Catholic experience to process it, even though my initial spiritual nurture as a Jesus-person was a *lectio divina* group in our Catholic parish. Her dismissive reaction closed a door between us, and the subject of spirituality was taboo for the next ten years, at least.

During that time I was discerning a call to the ministry and pursuing Presbyterian ordination. My need for Mom's love and respect was so intertwined with my spiritual life as to make it very difficult for me, in my twenties and thirties, to receive the love of God as affection. I felt God loved me because he had to, but not because he wanted to. This also summed up my struggles with Teresa of Ávila's *Interior Castle* the first time through.

Nevertheless, through the patient, gracious, good example of many members of the Christian community, not to mention my husband's incredible encouragement throughout our marriage, I eventually learned how to "be anxious for nothing" (Phil. 3:4–6). God generously provided me with other "mothers." My mother-in-law, Eleanor, was the primary, and after her death in 1998, mother figures among my friends, colleagues, and parishioners entered my life to show the calm way of trusting God. They all helped me to receive what God had so richly given—willingly and lavishly—and to know without doubt the height and depth of God's love.

The Catholic tradition often refers to "mother church." On any given Sunday morning, we are sisters and brothers in need of the demonstrative love of our Savior and Shepherd, Jesus Christ. The healing, remedial work that has been carried out both in, and now through, me has taken place in the fellowship of Christian disciples—"mother church," if you will.

In the end I can only be sad for the joys my mom was unable to experience, for the burdens of worry she carried needlessly, and for the roadblocks to relationships she erected to shelter herself from risk. Testifying to God's comfort and reassurance of a better way to live, my siblings and I picked the following Scripture for her memorial service:

> But now, thus says the Lord,
>> who created you, O Jacob, and formed
>> you, O Israel:
> Fear not, for I have redeemed you;
>> I have called you by name: you are mine.
> When you pass through the water, I will be with you;
>> in the rivers you shall not drown.
> When you walk through fire, you shall not be burned;
>> the flames shall not consume you.
> For I am the Lord, your God,
>> the Holy One of Israel, your savior.
> I give Egypt as your ransom,
>> Ethiopia and Seba in return for you.
> Because you are precious in my eyes
>> and glorious, and because I love you.
> (Isa. 43:1–4a)

135 ✒

My Mother, Myself: A Final Word

SATURDAY, APRIL 26, 2014

THE SKAGIT COUNTY TULIP FESTIVAL in Mount Vernon, Washington, draws crowds to view acres and acres of colorful bulbs each April. In the intervening days between my mother's death and her memorial Mass, my husband and daughter ventured forth to explore the tulip fields. The pair brought back two bouquets, knowing tulips are my favorite flower. I brought them to Mom's church the next day for her service. The reason I love the tulip is that it is the only flower that continues to grow after it is cut. A very tight, short arrangement of blooms grows gangly over time, but cutting the flower cannot stop its stem from developing further. I used this image at my mother's memorial Mass to illustrate the fact that she was a survivor.

This quality was tested most seriously upon the sudden death of her husband, my dad, at the age of sixty-eight in 1996. They had been married forty-three years, and Mom loved and depended on him as her rock of Gibraltar, protector, and provider. He experienced a brain hemorrhage while sitting at the dinner table one night and died the next day, on the Feast of the Epiphany. Mother's world crashed. It wasn't a matter of scary finances, for Mom had managed the family books for years and was well off. Rather, it was the loss of emotional support from a husband who had kept her at the center of his life and tried to protect her from the threats that caused her fear and anxiety. When he departed, her sense of security was shattered.

Over the next year or two, she worked through the initial crisis. She and Dad had researched suitable retirement communities in preparation for downsizing from the family home. She was on a waiting list for a senior housing cooperative, and when the right unit became available, she culled out their belongings, held an estate sale, and moved. There she made new friends and renewed fellowship with church and choir acquaintances. She even joined the board, serving a year as president. She contributed to the life of that community, and many of her friends shared their gratitude for her participation, calling her a "great lady."

Although my mom's issues spilled over into the next generation, she wanted to continue to grow. Evidence exists that this growth was focused primarily on internal, spiritual growth, to which her children were not necessarily privy while she lived. Going through her books, spiral notebooks, and even sneaking an unauthorized peak at key dates in her journal before it was taken away, I became aware that she was on a spiritual quest to anchor her soul in the stability and security only God could provide.

She has now run the race set before her and survived. The run wasn't always tidy, and she bumped a few walls and probably a few people along the path. But she crossed the finish line with a great cloud of witnesses surrounding her; among them, of course, was Dad (Heb. 12:1–3).

It may seem odd to say she survived her death, but in fact, as Christians we not only survive in this life, we survive the passage through death into new life in Christ. This is cause for great rejoicing, the fulfillment of the resurrection promise that in Christ, we too have been made alive. Mom is now completely at peace, without worry, without tears, without fear. God's perfect love poured into her soul has freed her from all of that. She is an overcomer.

Some years back she asked that a prayer be read to conclude her service. I strongly suspect that she wrote it herself, because I am sure she would have made an attribution if it had been penned by anyone else. It reveals the quest of her soul, and it has brought me great comfort in my own sorrow at her passing.

Finality

Lord, we are moving closer.

    Sometimes there is no gulf between us at all;

    and as I kneel before Your immensity, I dare to hope

        that I am also a tiny part of it.

    How relentlessly You have pursued me in spite of my waverings,

        in all settings and circumstances,

    forgiving my foolish attachments to false gods,

    overlooking my stubborn search for unchanging reality apart from You.

    But now I see that throughout my life

    I have needed only to walk with You at my side,

    that sooner or later everything else—people, places, memories—

        have needed to drop away.

    Only slowly have I seen that this dropping away of each created thing

    has given me time and space to move closer to You.

    Soon there will be no need for either faith or hope;

    at the end let only love remain, only love.

    Presently, I who have revered language will have no further need even for words.

    For at last, after so many lines and phrases, after countless questions and texts,

    I shall join You soon and forever, Lord, in Your own first language, silence.

136 🖋

Slept Away the Day

SATURDAY, APRIL 26, 2014, 4:20 A.M.

I HAVE BEEN GETTING SLEEPIER and sleepier as chemo round 4 has progressed. Yesterday my chemo infusion was pushed to the afternoon. This gave me an entire morning to wait out the nausea without "the good stuff" I usually receive in a morning IV drip. So I slept nearly all day and was so grateful for the rides, companionship, and cooking help of my friends to get me through it. Now it's 4:20 Saturday morning, and, as is typical on this crazy chemo schedule, I am perking up quite nicely, thank you.

I consulted with the medical oncologist yesterday afternoon: blood counts are virtually normal, and all is well. Just one more chemo treatment on Monday, and I am done with that phase. I want to bring a party to the cancer center on Monday, in celebration, so I'm thinking about what to bake in preparation.

On Wednesday the pulmonologist prescribed a new inhaler. It's a once-a-day dose, easy to use, and my pulmonary function numbers are already going up. We will step down from this to a corticosteroid in about six weeks, during which I hope to see marked improvement and greater stamina for exercise. It's hard to say what has caused the breathing difficulty, as my lung capacity is now normal—amazing lung volume. It's the bronchial airways that are constricted and inflamed, perhaps due in part to the epic allergy season we are experiencing. But if this new medicine works, not for much longer, I hope.

137 ✑

Done with Chemo!

MONDAY, APRIL 28, 2014, 4:58 P.M.

LAST CHEMO TREATMENT IS COMPLETE. The Beast is vanquished, dead, and buried. Nausea does not even rise to level of "queasy" today, though it will probably increase through the week. I am not afraid, though—just happy to be saying goodbye to toxins.

Since I felt too under the weather yesterday to bake anything, my friend Cindy brought her extra maple cupcakes for me to take to the infusion center for party time. As I left, I was invited to ring the bell—mounted on the wall for this celebratory purpose—at which point everybody in the center cheered my good fortune. It was a nice send-off. I plan on celebrating this date every year in gratitude.

Ongoing medical surveillance for the next three years includes blood work, imaging, and evaluation every three months.

My season of special need now ends. I believe we have seen the last of the Beast.

Gratitude wells up from the bottom of my heart for all those who have helped get me to this point. Now they get to witness the complete answer to prayer, my cure. Rejoice with me for the new lease on life God has given me. Let us all *live* joyfully to worship the Lord and serve his kingdom the rest of our days.

138 ✑

Normal vs. Transformed Life

TUESDAY, APRIL 29, 2014

ALENE KUDELA BURGERT WAS MY roommate during our senior year at Stanford. Our friendship has been renewed by visits in the last few years, most recently last summer in Bomet, Kenya, where she and husband Steve are missionaries.

Yesterday I received a handmade card from Alene. It touched me very deeply. On the cover is a rather fanciful elephant—known for its leisurely and silent tread across Africa's plains and forests—and the caption: "Hurry, hurry has no blessing. –African Proverb."

Alene's handwritten note expands on this proverb:

> Dear Andy and Mary,
>
> Prayers continue for you both as you go forward on your healing journey. It must seem slow on some days, but the Lord takes us slowly so we don't miss any of His blessings. He is not interested in "things getting back to normal," but [in] how this stage of the journey can bring us closer to conforming to the image of his Son. [If we go] too fast, we forget or miss the lessons. May the Lord continue His perfect and "perfecting" work in you both, even as He shapes us here in Kenya.
>
> Our gratitude . . . In his love and fellowship, Alene and Steve

Dallas Willard, similarly, was fond of insisting, "You must ruthlessly eliminate hurry from your life, for hurry is the great enemy of spiritual life in our world today."

Alene, as a chaplain in an African community, appreciates the slow-motion existence of my healing journey, in waiting rooms, chemo chairs, family room recliner, and ICU. Not to mention the monotonous routines for self-maintenance and pulmonary rehabilitation following surgery, which require slow, deep breathing and a balance between getting sufficient air and intensity of exercise.

During the last six months, my journal has expressed in slow-motion the unfolding story of God's love for me through lung cancer, enriched friendships, unknowns, then knowns, victories, discouragements, and the death of my mother. Is it coincidence that these narrative arcs have coincided with the flow of the church year? Themes from Advent to Easter have guided my reflections on what God was and is saying and doing within my soul.

But now I have passed a milestone; this part of the journey is coming to an end. Yesterday was my last chemo treatment. From here forward, I am building up strength and stamina and setting what I hope will be a fairly uninterrupted trajectory toward new and renewed life goals.

It seems appropriate to look at my expectations for life in the Before Cancer days in mid-August 2013 and to see how life's river has tumbled over rocks and logjams into the pool of new life I now enjoy. I am choosing between forks in the river—renewal of pastoral ministry or perhaps retirement?—but doing so without hurry in order not to miss God's blessing, Jesus's voice, and the Holy Spirit's power for the moment and for the future.

So thank you, Alene, for such a lovely note that encourages my mind and heart toward the future God would have for me. Thank you for the reminder that our goal is not normal life but transformed life. The question going forward has become, What is the new normal for which God has prepared my soul and body?

139 🍃

The Dynamic of Reassigned Duty

Wednesday, April 30, 2014

In my Before Cancer days, professional life was directed to four main areas: serving part time as an interim pastoral associate at a large Lutheran church, serving as executive director of a national organization, coordinating the evangelical caucus of my presbytery, and teaching at a multidenominational seminary. I had served as a pastor in two church families from 1987 through 2006, and the transition from parish pastor to freelance minister at large in 2007 was a major adjustment of identity and work style. Since then I have experienced several transitions, becoming practiced at leaving the old and embracing the new. Well, actually, keeping the old and adding the new. It would have been accurate to refer to "the nine [simultaneous] lives of Mary Naegeli." I am exhausted just thinking about the pace I maintained in those decades.

All that changed on November 4, 2013, when I was diagnosed with lung cancer and began an aggressive treatment plan. The phrase that describes my transition best is "a reassignment of duty," or what the Navy calls "temporary additional duty." This is the watchword that has stuck with my friends, because it is what I shared with my congregation when I found out what was happening last fall. "I've been reassigned duty, and I will embrace my new call with the same enthusiasm I have given serving you here at church." In the After Diagnosis era, I have been on leave at church, have delegated most organizational responsibilities, have been absent from presbytery meetings since last fall, and have bowed out of seminary teaching. Wow. That is quite a pruning! And yet, I have not felt these changes as losses as much as I have felt the vigorous calling to a new assignment.

From a biblical point of view, calling to a new assignment is frequently how God works. Among the notables, we have Abraham (Gen. 12) called from out of nowhere to become the father of a great nation. Then there is Joseph (Gen. 37–50), thrown into an empty cistern by his jealous brothers, only to be carted off to Egypt to become a country leader. Moses, of course (Exodus 3), was called out of shepherding to lead the Hebrews to the promised land. What all episodes have in common is that God picked somebody seemingly at random and said, "I've got a new job for you. I will lead you and help you, and it's going to be amazing and also hard."

As God says to me, "Mary Naegeli, I have a new job for you after cancer," anticipation rises in my heart. My illness invited me to reexamine my life, priorities, calling, and service. As a result of the growth process God orchestrated, change no longer poses a threat to my soul or self-image. I have the freedom and the inner strength to choose a quieter life, if that is what God requires. I will have greater physical strength and stamina if God returns me to wider responsibility. Whatever unfolds, my life is in God's hands.

I have learned a transforming lesson. No matter how steep or difficult the path, if I breathe deeply of God's Spirit, I can remain calm. Even through cancer, Jesus Christ has proven himself trustworthy, and his love is wide and deep and secure.

EPILOGUE

A Prayer (with Seven Deep Breaths)

L OVING GOD,

1
We breathe in your life,
knowing that in our stories of creation
your breath is our breath.
We breathe out our anxiety,
acknowledging the stress that increases
with every blaring headline and dire prediction.

2
We breathe in your hope,
knowing that you can make a way
out of no way.
We breathe out the despondency,
that creeps upon us,
paralyzing us from doing good.

3
We breathe in your grace,
as we pray for patience with our loved ones
and endurance in our sheltering.

We breathe out our petty annoyances,
and menial irritations
that make us forget the importance of our bonds.

4

We breathe in your peace,
which surpasses all our understanding,
and guards our hearts and minds.
We breathe out our worries,
all of our need to be in control,
and the tension in our guts.

5

We breathe in your abundance,
knowing that we have enough
when we live as a beloved community.
We breathe out our fear of scarcity,
that whispers lies to us
and keeps our fists clenched in greed.

6

We breathe in your wisdom,
that keeps perspective in our crisis,
reminding us of what is important.
We breathe out despair
that blocks us from seeing possibilities
and blinds us from your vision.

7

We breathe in your love,
knowing that your presence surrounds us,
and encircles us.
We breathe out the suffering
acknowledging that our pain happens
within your loving embrace.

—Carol Howard Merritt, written during the global pandemic of 2020

ACKNOWLEDGMENTS

MOST OF THE DATED ENTRIES first appeared in my blog *Bringing the Word to Life* at the time events were happening, and wrangling them into book form was no small feat. I am so grateful to friend Craig Pynn, himself a cancer survivor, who thoroughly edited my first draft and challenged this "thinker" to express her feelings. Editor Amanda Bird put her discerning mark on the manuscript, pointing out corrections and suggestions with heart and tact. Writing mentors at the Mount Hermon Christian Writers Conference, including Janet McHenry, Renae Brumbaugh Green, and Joseph Bentz, propelled my work forward. Thank you all for investing time and interest in this project. Thanks to my cousin, William DeJong, PhD, who wouldn't let me give up and showed me a way forward.

Thanks to Redemption Press for picking up this project, especially to Athena Dean Holtz for recognizing a story that will help many people and to Hannah McKenzie and Dori Harrell for giving steady hands to production of *Deep Breathing*.

Throughout my cancer experience, one thought entertained and humbled me: thousands of people were behind the success of my treatment—lab workers, pharmacists, engineers, doctors, pathologists, and scientists at the forefront of technological advance. The faces of this "great cloud of witnesses" were my personal cancer medical team, including doctors Gigi Chen (medical oncologist), Sophia Rahman (radiation oncologist), Michaela Straznicka (surgeon), Kristina Kramer (pulmonologist), and my primary care physician, Paul Endo. I am indebted to them and grateful to God for using them all so effectively in my case. Special thanks go to Dr. Rahman for reading my manuscript for medical accuracy and to Dr. Chen for pointing me toward helpful patient resources. But if by chance an error has slipped through, I alone bear responsibility.

Deep gratitude goes to my husband, Andy, who loved me through the lung cancer experience and supported the birthing of this book. Many thanks to daughter Judy for being a sounding board and consultant on all matters to do with writing, editing, and the World Wide Web, and to daughter Katy for being there at crucial moments on the journey.

PATIENT AND CAREGIVER RESOURCES

Lotsa Helping Hands: Care Calendar Website at https://lotsahelping-hands.com/.

Lotsa Helping Hands powers online caring communities that help restore health and balance to caregivers' lives. Its service brings together caregivers and volunteers through online communities that organize daily life during times of medical crisis or caregiver exhaustion.

Calendar-based and completely adaptable to your particular situation, the site is a helpful tool for coordinating all those people who have said to you, "Call me if you need anything."

GO2 Foundation for Lung Cancer at https://go2foundation.org/.

Founded by patients and survivors, GO_2 **Foundation for Lung Cancer** transforms survivorship as the world's leading organization dedicated to saving, extending, and improving the lives of those vulnerable, at risk, and diagnosed with lung cancer. The organization is working to change the reality of living with lung cancer by ending stigma, increasing public and private research funding, and ensuring access to care.

American Cancer Society patient resources at https://www.cancer.org/cancer/lung-cancer.html.

An excellent tutorial on the basics of lung cancer types, staging, and treatment. The survival statistics are available but buried in this site, so for those like me who would rather not get discouraged by numbers, you can orient to the lung cancer world and lingo with reliable information.

American Society of Clinical Oncology patient resources at https:// www.cancer.net/.

ASCO develops and publishes clinical practice guidelines, provisional clinical opinions (PCOs), and guideline endorsements, providing evidence-based recommendations to serve as a guide for doctors and outline appropriate methods of treatment and care. Its patient resources site www.cancer.net offers a range of information, navigational tools, and coping strategies for persons diagnosed, treated, or surviving cancers of all types. Special tabs for lung cancer are included.

BIBLIOGRAPHY

Ashbrook, R. Thomas. *Mansions of the Heart: Exploring the Seven Stages of Spiritual Growth*. San Francisco: Jossey-Bass, 2009.

Becker, Ernest. *The Denial of Death*. New York: Simon & Schuster, 1973.

Carretto, Carlo. *The Desert in the City*. London: Collins, 1979.

Covey, Stephen R. *The 7 Habits of Highly Effective People: Powerful Lessons in Personal Change*. New York: Fireside/Simon & Schuster, 1989.

Jones, E. Stanley. *Abundant Living*. Nashville: Abingdon, 1942, 1970.

Jones, E. Stanley. *The Divine Yes*. Nashville: Abingdon, 1963.

Kolodiejchuk, M.C., Brian. *Mother Teresa: Come Be My Light*. New York: Doubleday, 2007.

Kübler-Ross, Elisabeth. *On Death and Dying: What the Dying Have to Teach Doctors, Nurses, Clergy and Their Own Families*. New York: Scribner & Sons, 1969.

Lewis, C. S. *The Screwtape Letters*. New York: HarperCollins, 2001.

Lewis, C. S. *The Silver Chair*. New York: HarperCollins, 1953, 1981.

Thielicke, Helmut. *The Evangelical Faith*. 2 vols. Grand Rapids, MI: Wm. B. Eerdmans, 1974.

Willard, Dallas. *The Divine Conspiracy: Rediscovering Our Hidden Life in God*. San Francisco: HarperSanFrancisco, 1998.

Willard, Dallas. *Renovation of the Heart: Putting on the Character of Christ*. Colorado Springs: NavPress, 2002.

Wright, N. T. *Surprised by Hope: Rethinking Heaven, the Resurrection, and the Mission of the Church*. New York: HarperOne/HarperCollins, 2008.

Yadegaran, Jessica. "Death Café: Coffee, Cake & Grave Conversation." *Contra Costa Times*, January 15, 2014.

Order Information

REDEMPTION
P R E S S

To order additional copies of this book, please visit
www.redemption-press.com.
Also available on Amazon.com and BarnesandNoble.com
or by calling toll-free 1-844-2REDEEM.